Chronic Back Pain Solved

The Cause and Cure of Chronic Back Pain

GREG LARKIN

Copyright © 2018. All rights reserved.

This book, or parts thereof, may not be reproduced in any form without the written permission from the author; exceptions are made for brief excerpts used in publication reviews.

Printed in the United States of America

10 9 8 7 6 5 4 3 2

EMPIRE PUBLISHING

www.empirebookpublishing.com

Illustrator: Christian Deocampo
Website: www.christiandeocampo.com
Email: cdeodesign@gmail.com

Editor: Diane Eaton
Website: www.dianethewritingdoctor.com
Email: diane@dianethewritingdoctor.com

Table of Contents

Introduction i

Chapter 1 1

The First Eight Years 1

    Year One: First Injury 2

    Year One: Second Injury 7

    Year Two 16

    Year Three 20

    Year Four 23

    Year Five 26

    Year Six 29

    Year Seven 32

    Year Eight 34

Chapter 2 38

The Second Eight Years 38

    Year Nine 38

    Year Ten 39

    Year Eleven 41

    Year Twelve 44

    Year Thirteen 47

    Year Fourteen 47

    Year Fifteen 48

Year Sixteen..49

Chapter 3...51

Baby Steps 51

Anatomical Short Leg 52

Non-Anatomical Short Leg 52

Larkin Lift..57

Chapter 4...60

Chiropractic Care 60

Subluxation Pain 64

Types of Neurological Pain..68

Chapter 5...70

A Structural Analysis 70

Loaded vs. Unloaded Spine 74

Chapter 6...76

PRP..76

First Injections...77

Second Injections 77

More Injections 79

Neck Injections 81

Yet More Injections 82

Chapter 7...86

Ligament Laxity 86

Extra Amount 89

Why Was This Not Diagnosed? 90

Chapter 8 92

Muscle Imbalance 92

    Stuck States 95

Chapter 9 96

The Larkin Method 96

    Step 1 – Correct Subluxations 97

    Step 2 – Modify Posture 98

    Step 3 – Loosen and Lengthen Muscles...................................99

    Step 4 – Repair Ligaments 102

    Step 5 – Correct Muscle Imbalance 103

    Your Insurance Isn't Enough 105

Chapter 10 106

The Real Solution 106

    Proof Positive 114

Chapter 11 115

Our Healthcare System 115

    Why No Scientific Evidence Supporting Chiropractic Care Exists 118

Chapter 12 121

Why Chiropractors Get No Respect 121

    Flaws of Chiropractic Care 122

    The Solution 124

Chapter 13 126

How Physical Therapy Gets It All Wrong 126

    The Physical Therapy Treatment Model 129

Chapter 14 132

    Categories of People 132

        Category 1 132

        Category 2 132

        Category 3 133

        Category 4 134

        Something in Common 135

Chapter 15 138

    Other People With Chronic Back Pain 138

Chapter 16 145

    I Can Ruin Anyone's Life 145

        No Takers 149

Chapter 17 151

    How Did I Get Here? 151

        Orthopedic Surgeons 153

        Why Did I Have to Solve This Problem? 155

        How To Solve Chronic Back Pain 157

        I Did It My Way 158

        Starting the Conversation 159

Chapter 18 162

    Living pain free 162

Chronic Back Pain Solved

Introduction

This is the story of my journey through life with debilitating, chronic back pain—and my work to find a real solution that would allow me to live without it.

It's a story that I would rather not tell, but I feel I must. It's important to me to share with you several things I've learned from my journey: how chronic back pain develops, what I endured as I tried to find solutions, and the methods I finally used to solve my back pain problem once and for all. Armed with this information, you benefit from my journey and learn how to free yourself from pain.

My goal with this book is to fundamentally change the way our healthcare system currently treats chronic back pain. There are way too many people who are living and suffering with it. If I can prove the current treatment model is wrong, I can help these people. If I can help just one person get out of chronic pain, then all of the time that I have spent searching for answers, documenting results, and writing this book will have been worth it. I am confident that, if my ideas are actually implemented, millions of people can be helped in very real ways.

I believe that the information I provide in this book is worth billions of dollars. That's right, billions with a "b". If you add up all of the people who are suffering with chronic panic and then figure out the cumulative financial cost of dealing with it, the numbers are staggering. Between medical costs, lost wages, and out-of-pocket expenses, my financial costs were in the millions of dollars. The financial toll of chronic back pain is a huge burden on society and someone has to pay for it.

For many, many years, I lived with brutal chronic pain in my back. If you've experienced chronic pain, you know that you'd try almost anything and spend whatever you need to spend if it means you might reduce the pain. Over the course of these many years, I saw a vast number of doctors and medical specialists, and I have spent a lot of money. I saw almost every type of practitioner available and I have had more procedures done on me than I can count. I went to doctor after doctor seeking answers and letting them do whatever they could do to give me relief from my pain. If they recommended a specialist, I went to see them, too. I've been to physical therapists, chiropractors, massage therapists, pain medicine specialists, and orthopedic surgeons. I've spent many hours doing massage, acupuncture, traction, yoga, and fascial stretching. I'd see pretty much anyone who promised me any degree of pain relief.

This book documents the systematic approach I used to rid myself of my chronic back pain. I started by trying to learn what the cause of my pain was. I then applied a step-by-step approach to solve problem after problem until I came up with a solution. What I uncovered through this process is extraordinary. I now understand why so many people live with chronic pain and why they will live with it until they die. Once you read this, you will, too.

I decided to take a scientific approach to solving the riddle of my chronic back pain. I am an electronics engineer, a scientist in effect, and as such, I chose to approach my problem using the scientific method. The scientific method is widely accepted as the gold standard for providing explanations about why something behaves in a certain way. Scientists use it to acquire new knowledge or to correct what has been previously concluded about a subject.

The scientific method consists of a set of four steps that anyone can follow to reach a conclusion. The first step consists of asking a question. The second step entails developing a hypothesis, a proposed explanation to the question or problem. The third step consists of collecting data to support the hypothesis. This can be accomplished using a variety of methods like experimentation or observation. The final step of the scientific method consists of drawing a conclusion.

When I applied the scientific method to determine the cause of chronic back pain, I came up with the following:

Step 1: The Question

Here was my question: *Why are millions of people living with chronic back pain?*

I needed to answer that question for myself so I could understand why—or if—I had to live with chronic back pain every day of my life. And I knew I was not alone. There are millions of people who are living with chronic back pain in this country. I needed to know why no one was helping any of us to find a real solution.

Step 2: The Hypothesis

Here was my hypothesis: *The current method for treating chronic back pain is fundamentally flawed.*

My hypothesis was that the reason people continue to suffer from chronic back pain is that no one in medicine understands the true cause of chronic back pain. Therefore; they do not know how to treat it.

Step 3: Gather Data

To answer Question 1, I was very methodical as I went searching for the answer to chronic back pain. I gathered a lot of data over sixteen years, which I share with you in this book. I present a ton of information that will show you how I came to confirm my hypothesis that the current method for treating chronic back pain is fundamentally flawed.

Step 4: Draw a Conclusion

The conclusion I drew is presented in this book. As you read, you'll discover that most people with chronic back pain share similar issues. You'll be shown the data that proves that chronic back pain is a solvable problem and that people don't need to live with it until they die.

By proving that my hypothesis is correct, I prove that everyone in medicine who is treating chronic back pain—and not getting results—is wrong. I prove that every physical therapist is wrong. Every orthopedic surgeon is wrong. Every pain medicine specialist is wrong. Every chiropractor is sort of wrong. My job is to present the information.

Your job is to draw your own conclusion armed with the stories, reports, and information I present in this book. If you suffer from chronic back pain, I believe it can make a huge difference for you as you find the solutions for yourself.

Chapter 1
The First Eight Years

Pain is somewhat subjective; people experience it with different levels of intensity and response. If a bee stings you, the pain is very intense at first, but it goes away quickly. While the pain level you experience from a sting may be very high, the overall disturbance of your quality of life is probably minimal. With chronic pain, on the other hand, the pain itself might be anything from mild to very intense; but either way, it is constant. As such, it impacts your quality of life.

Relentless pain inevitably starts to wear on you and takes over your life. It affects you physically and emotionally. It limits what you can do in your life, it can require you to make major lifestyle changes, and it can cause you increasing levels of stress and suffering.

I make this point because, even if the pain you're feeling at any particular time is not too bad, if it's a chronic condition over which you have no control, your quality of life can sink to very low levels. So, to convey the full experience of my journey with chronic back pain, I refer to what I call a Quality of Life (QOL) scale in this book. It ranges from 1 to 10, where 10 indicates that I'm experiencing absolutely no pain and my quality of life could hardly get any better. On the other hand, a 1 on the QOL scale signifies that I'm in chronic pain, and emotionally, I'm hitting the wall. If I were to ever get to 0 on the QOL scale, I'd pretty much take my own life.

Before I started living with chronic pain in my back, I was a diehard athlete. Anything that gave me a great workout and left me drenched in sweat, I absolutely loved. I loved to go to the gym and I loved to get together with my friends to enjoy outdoor sports. I loved playing tennis. For me, as long as the weather was halfway decent, it was tennis weather. I lived in Denver, Colorado, where the weather might start out nice enough to play tennis but by the time we were done, it would be snowing. It didn't matter as far as we were concerned. I lived in tennis shorts because I was playing so much. If I wasn't playing tennis, then I was mountain biking, skiing, or hiking. Mountain biking often meant riding up a mountain for a couple thousand feet so my friends and I could enjoy the ride back down. When we skied, it was mogul or powder skiing all day long.

We were diehards who weren't afraid of marathon days. We might start out playing tennis for three or four hours, then eat some lunch, then move onto mountain biking, then stop to eat some dinner. We'd finish out the day at the gym and eat again. We were burning a lot of calories. I was in exceptionally good physical shape and I enjoyed it.

Then one day, everything changed.

Year One: First Injury

It was August when some friends of mine asked me to join them in a game of roller hockey. I had never been on rollerblades before and I found them surprisingly hard to get used to, even for an experienced athlete like myself. Playing the sport was just a little awkward. After all, you have to bend forward while swinging a stick at the same time, which isn't a natural or easy thing to do. As I learned the sport, I could feel my lower back muscles working hard, but I figured I was a big strong guy and I could handle it.

After a round of roller hockey one afternoon, I felt something wasn't quite right with my back. It had tightened up and the pain in my upper back would not go away. I don't remember any particular incident that seemed to be the culprit, causing the pain. I hadn't had any major collisions with anyone; I hadn't fallen on the ground, or hit any object. There was no blood. At first, I figured I just pulled a muscle or something. Never having dealt with that type of pain before, it started to get really annoying. It was just enough pain to make me want to stop all activities and sit on the couch. It wasn't long until I had to take some time off of work to rest my back. But after a couple of days of rest, I realized that the pain wasn't going away any time soon. I had to see someone and get some help.

I decided to go see my general physician. He gave me a quick examination and an X-Ray. The doctor placed me on an intersegmental table that had rollers that moved up and down my spine to try to realign my spine. The theory was that maybe something in my back was simply out of alignment. I remember thinking, *My back is killing me and you want me to lie on this stupid table? This is all you are going to do for me? Seriously, help me please!*

The general physician didn't recommend that I see a chiropractor or physical therapist. His approach was to tell me to "give it a little time" and see if maybe the pain would just go away. He didn't prescribe any medications, but recommended that I see an orthopedic surgeon.

I walked out of his office feeling pretty depressed. After all, he hadn't given me any solutions to my agonizing problem. It dawned on me that, first, he had no clue what was wrong with me and, second, he wasn't able to help me. Unfortunately, it would not be the last time that I worked with someone who had no answers for me.

I had just purchased a house and had recently started a new job. I had bills to pay. I couldn't just stop working for a while and see how things improved. I considered myself a pretty tough guy, so I decided to just deal with the pain and hope it would go away soon. I stopped all physical activities and just tried to make it through each day. For someone like myself, working out and getting exercise was a big part of my life. They were my stress relievers and sources of great enjoyment. Being in pain was hard; but not being able to exercise was brutal.

It took some time to actually get in to see the orthopedic surgeon, but the day finally arrived. We had a brief chat and I told him where my pain was. He performed his physical exam and moved me into a variety of positions to see if he could recreate my pain. None of the movements caused any significant pain. He took an X-Ray, which didn't reveal anything obvious. He gave me no explanation of I was in pain. He ordered an MRI and sent me on my way.

Of course, things take time. It took a week to do the MRI. I then had to schedule a follow-up appointment with the orthopedic surgeon, and that took another week. I was stuck living in pain day after day. I continued to work and hoped the MRI would help us learn what the problem was.

When I returned to the orthopedic surgeon, he told me that he had reviewed my MRI and found no issues. He didn't recommend surgery and he gave me no other options. On one hand, it felt like a huge relief because he saw nothing that required a surgery. I had heard horror stories about people who have failed back surgery. On the other hand, it was a huge let down because I had not been given a plan to get better. The doctor didn't recommend that I see a physical therapist or chiropractor. He didn't prescribe any muscle relaxants or painkillers. I walked out of his office thinking, *Here is another person who is not going to help me. He had no clue what was wrong with me.*

I was stuck. I was living in pain day after day and I was given no explanation of why it was happening. I was pretty depressed. The pain felt like a constant ache and was intense enough that I decided to stop doing anything beyond walking and sitting. Still, the pain wasn't bad enough for me to leave work and file for disability. My muscles had become very tight. I would have to take a hot bath at the end of the day just to get a little relief. I tried to resume my life and just accept the pain. Over time, I started to experience some very small improvements in the pain level. Or maybe I just got used to living with it.

A few months later, I went on a camping trip to a location that was about five hours away from my home. While I was there, I got on a four-wheeler and immediately felt a jolt of intense pain in my upper back. I stayed at the camp that night and tried to see if the pain would calm down on its own. I was in so much pain that I couldn't even sleep through the night. I got in my car to drive the five hours to get home, but after about two and half hours, I realized I couldn't go on. I took myself to the Emergency Room in Glenwood Springs, Colorado. They found nothing wrong with my back and I was given painkillers so that I could continue my trip. After a few days, the pain had calmed down a little and I returned to work.

As a part of my job, I occasionally traveled to Singapore for a month at a time. The trip from Denver to Singapore entailed a very long plane ride—24 hours door to door. Since I was fairly new at the company, refusing to go was not an option for me.

The plane ride was somewhat painful, but the pain was manageable and I was able to get through it without painkillers. I felt relieved just to be able to get there in one piece. The second I got to my hotel, I soaked in the tub.

Within a few days, I felt like going to the gym at the hotel to see if I could loosen up my muscles a little bit. When I got there, one of my coworkers was there lifting weights and he asked me to spot him while he was doing bench presses. I told him that my back was hurting me and I was not sure if I should spot someone. I was halfway around the world and the last thing I needed was more back pain.

The job of a spotter varies widely depending upon the person being spotted. Some people just need a little assistance and will push through the entire exercise, giving it all they have. Other people give up more quickly and expect their spotter to lift the weight after they've reached their limit, with no help from them. Spotting someone doing a bench press meant that I would be bent forward while trying to lift a heavy weight—not a very back-friendly activity.

The guy told me it would be a light spot so I said okay. I remember thinking, *Are you sure you want to do this?* Turns out I needed to exert much more force than I thought I'd need to. I was bent over trying to place a bar back on the rack, thinking, *What are you doing? He lied to me!*

Then, I heard a pop in my back. I was startled. The last thing I wanted to do was to injure my back, even just a little bit. I thought for sure that I was screwed. But once I calmed down, I discovered that my back wasn't any worse. In fact, from that point on, it seemed to be pain-free.

For the rest of my time in Singapore, I felt a lot better and seemed to have no limitations. I returned to living a normal and surprisingly pain-free life. The flight back was no problem, and once at home, I resumed every activity that I used to do. I did everything that I wanted to do with no pain. The pain had miraculously disappeared.

It was October. I had endured about two months of debilitating pain but my ordeal and torturous journey seemed to be over. Finally, I was feeling like my old self again: young and healthy. My quality of life had skyrocketed from a 4 to a 10 and I thought the worst was behind me.

I was wrong.

Year One: Second Injury

The next several months continued pretty uneventfully. I was back at skiing, lifting weights, mountain biking, and playing tennis. I had no pain and I had no health issues. In fact, I was feeling so good that I decided to try roller hockey again. Now I know that might sound like an obviously bad idea, but I felt really strong and I just didn't think it would be a problem. Besides, I had a whole lot of roller hockey gear in my car that I had spent a lot of money on. Might as well get some good use out of it, right?

I was enjoying getting back into the game again but within a few weeks I started to notice a problem. I started feeling some pain in my lower back from being bent over while swinging a stick. I was a poor skater and it was hurting me, not helping me. The better skaters around me seemed to skate in more of an upright position.

Even though my back started to feel a little stiff, I decided to keep playing. I figured that some activity might be a good idea; maybe it would help loosen my back up. One day, I had a light collision with another player, but there was no incident to speak of. I didn't fall down and there was no blood. But by the time the game was over, my lower back was in a lot of pain. I had been there before and it scared me. I didn't want to go back into the pain cycle I knew much too well.

I went back to work that day, but my back pain was so severe that I took the rest of the day off to relax. My home was about a half-hour drive from work and I spent every minute of the drive in excruciating pain. I couldn't get any relief except by lying in a certain position on the couch; I couldn't even stand up. At that point, my quality of life sunk pretty low. I'd call it a 1.

After spending the weekend lying on my back, the pain abated slightly. The following Monday, I went back to work, still in pain, but able to get some things done. I was a fighter.

It was obvious to me that I needed to see an orthopedic surgeon again. As usual, it took time to get on their schedule, so I waited. In pain once more, this time the wait was much worse. Just trying to make it through the day took all of my energy. I couldn't do anything; even standing and sitting were incredibly hard.

The pain was in a different place than it had been before—it was in my lower back. So the orthopedic surgeon decided he wanted me to get another MRI. Now, I had been through the ordeal before: I'd count the days until the MRI and then I'd count the days until I could see the orthopedic surgeon again. Every day was sheer hell. I prayed that he had a solution to make it all worth it.

When I finally got in to see him, he looked at my MRI and diagnosed me with degenerative disc disease in the lowest two segments of my back. He told me that degenerative disc disease occurs when a disc has become degraded, including a loss of spacing and a loss of fluid. It's easy to spot degenerative disc disease on an MRI because the discs are darker than the other discs. Since he didn't see any obvious disc bulges compressing my nerves, he told me that I didn't need surgery. There was nothing else of note on my MRI, he said.

Even though he gave me a diagnosis, the surgeon couldn't tell me what was causing my back pain and he offered no solution to make it go away. From my perspective, the only good news was that whatever was causing the pain was not serious enough to require a surgery. He prescribed muscle relaxants for me and told me to go see a physical therapist.

I walked out of this doctor's office for the second time, without any answers about how to help reduce my debilitating back pain. But at least I now had a name for what might be the cause of my pain: degenerative disc disease. I researched the condition diligently. The strange thing is that the statistics show that a large number of people have the disease but it has never been directly linked to any cause of pain. Some people have pain and some people don't. It was not quite the slam-dunk of a diagnosis that I was hoping for. I did learn that the discs don't have a good blood supply so, once injured, they don't heal easily on their own. I realized I might have to live with the disease until I died.

Once again, my company told me they wanted me to do some work in Singapore and I felt I had to go or I could lose my job. I had a little time before I was scheduled to leave, so I went to see a physical therapist. The therapist listened to my story and did a physical examination. She gave me the impression that she was new to her job or was acting as an assistant, treating me as if I had a pulled muscle in my back. She performed ultrasound and massage and gave me some basic exercises that she said were going to strengthen the muscles around my spine. I saw her for a couple of visits but didn't experience any pain relief at all. With my first incident, my back pain had just suddenly gone away on its own. I was hoping it might do the same thing again this time.

I was very nervous about the trip to Singapore because of the extreme pain I was in. I could barely sit down and I'd have to stand up frequently just to get a little pain relief. It was going to be a very long trip. I wasn't sure if I could endure the limousine ride to the airport, let alone a flight halfway around the world. I was not even convinced that I could carry my own bag through the airport. What happens if the pain were to get worse? Could I find the help I needed in Singapore? Would I be able to get back home?

I stocked up on painkillers and muscle relaxants. While I considered myself a strong person, I was scared to death. And the stress was brutal.

I could only put off the trip for so long, so I packed my bags and prepared to leave the country. Turns out that the limousine driver had back issues, so we started talking. He had seven levels of vertebrae fused together and he was relatively pain-free. He was able to lift his passengers' heavy bags and sit in his limousine for hours at a time. He gave me some hope that, if I had fusion surgery, the outcome might be positive. My life might return to normal.

Once the plane bound for Singapore took off, I started to calm down a little bit and think things through a little more. I was doing what I had to do, going to Singapore and sticking it out as best as I could. I might lose one month of my life to painkillers, I thought, but I was going to keep my job all right.

The plane ride was miserable. The moment I got settled in the hotel, I got in the tub to soak my back for some pain relief. I was in a foreign country halfway around the world and in miserable pain. *What the hell was I thinking?*

I worked very long days in Singapore and it was very hard for me to endure the pain I was experiencing. I was taking muscle relaxants three times a day and they made me very tired. I tried to do the exercises that the physical therapist had recommended but they were too aggressive and ended up causing me even more pain. The only thing that provided any relief was a hot bath every night. I would say that my QOL was on life-support at a 0.5 at that point. I could hardly get any lower and still be breathing.

I couldn't wait for the trip to be over; I was exhausted from being stressed out, overworked, and in constant pain. The drawback was that I knew I had a very long plane ride home—but it was worth it. I took my muscle relaxants and flew home. Once I got back, I was very tired, but the comfort of being in my own home was incredible. My quality of life climbed all the way up to a 1. It had been one miserable journey.

I still had hope that I might be able to find someone who could help me. So I went back to the physical therapist and started doing more exercises, including using a Swiss ball and going swimming. I'd do the therapy at lunch but I didn't really feel like it was doing me any good. My muscle spasms were still painful and I couldn't sit down for very long.

The pain was flaring up even when I was just engaged in normal activities but, over time, it slowly calmed down and I started feeling a little better. I returned to the gym to do very light workouts. One day, I thought I was feeling well enough to hit some tennis balls. Unfortunately, I learned very quickly that it was a huge mistake. For hours afterward, I was on the floor in horrible pain.

I started to recognize that I couldn't do any of the activities that I used to do. The money had run out for physical therapy, so that ended that. I continued to do exercises on my own but I seemed to get no benefit from it. I tried weaning myself off of the muscle relaxants but I found that my muscles tightened up so fast that I death-spiraled back into horrible pain. I had to stay on the muscle relaxants.

When I decided to go back to see my orthopedic surgeon, my girlfriend wanted to come along. She was tired of seeing me suffer in pain all the time and she wanted some answers for herself. She put together a list of questions to ask him:

1. On a physical level, what is happening when Greg is in pain compared to when he is feeling good?
2. Six months ago, he seemed to have made a full recovery and he had no pain. Yet, according to the diagnosis, he had the degenerative discs then. How is that possible?

3. What will be the physical difference in his back between how it is now, when he's in pain, and after a full recovery some months down the road, in light of the fact that the degenerative disc will never regenerate?

4. If he makes a full recovery will the degenerative disc disease go away?

5. What causes the muscle spasms? Are they a sign of healing? Are they a sign he has pushed it too far? What is the best treatment for spasms?

6. As you've indicated, Greg has apparently had the degenerative disc disease for several years. What is the injury he suffered on the day he played roller hockey? Did he pinch the nerve? Damage or tear muscle? Displace the disc? Tear something else? As I understand, Degenerative Disc Disease is a slow process and couldn't happen in a sudden movement. What physically happened in the sudden movement of roller hockey to cause all of Greg's pain?

7. What can be done in the future to prevent the disc from further degeneration and to prevent other discs from beginning to degenerate?

8. Is degeneration hereditary? Is it linked to a mineral deficiency? Is it a posture problem?

9. Are stretches a good idea? Is the muscle injured? Would weekly massages help? Would using a heating pad for several hours a day help to reduce the pain?

My girlfriend was just as frustrated as I was that no one was helping me reduce my torturous pain. But we never got an answer to any of these questions. I honestly think that the surgeon didn't know how to answer them. He didn't know what was wrong with me and he didn't want to take the time to tell me that.

The orthopedic surgeon told me I only had a few options to try and get some relief from the pain I was experiencing every day. One was to have spinal fusion surgery. Due to the severity of my disease, I would need a two-level spinal fusion surgery, which would mean removing two discs and inserting a metal cage in my back. But I've heard horror stories of people who have had fusion surgeries. The statistics said that the chance of having a successful fusion was very low so I was pessimistic that it would do me any good. Besides, I really didn't want to remove my discs on some slim chance that it might solve my problem.

The only other option I had was to go to a pain medicine specialist, who would prescribe a variety of medications, including painkillers. I had decided not to take any pain medication at the time. I had heard about people who were addicted to painkillers and I had no interest in going down that path unless I was absolutely desperate.

So from my perspective, I really had no options. I could have surgery that offers a very low success rate or I could start taking pain medication and hope that I don't become an addict. I didn't want either. It was very depressing for me to have no choices. So I just continued on, one horrible day after the next.

A few months later, my insurance started over and I was able to see a physical therapist again. I was having a lot of pain in my pelvis and the lower right side of my back. Ultrasound provided a small amount of temporary relief but I started feeling a tingling pain in my legs that no one had any answers for. The orthopedic surgeon had recommended that I see a chiropractor, so I stopped seeing the physical therapist and started seeing the chiropractor. I had absolutely no idea what they did, but I would do anything for some pain relief.

The chiropractor took an X-Ray of my back and determined that my degenerative disk disease was very minor and probably was not causing my pain. When he reviewed my MRI, he said he didn't see anything that would cause any alarm. I saw him for a couple of weeks and I didn't notice any improvement. Once again, it was obvious that this professional was not going to help me. So I stopped seeing him.

I started experiencing nausea, so I had to stop taking the muscle relaxants for a while. I had a blood test taken just to make sure everything was normal. I went to see a second orthopedic surgeon, I showed him my MRI, and we discussed all of my problems. He did his own evaluation and decided that he couldn't do anything to reduce my pain. I found it ironic that while I passed his physical evaluation with flying colors, I'd be in more pain than usual for weeks afterwards. He recommended that I see a physical therapist or a chiropractor. I have been down that rat hole before and I wasn't interested in revisiting it.

Emotionally, I sank lower and lower each time I sought help only to hear that they didn't know how to reduce my pain.

I was in so much pain that I had no choice but to see another physical therapist. This one recommended that I try using orthotics in my shoes. I was not sure how orthotics could possibly help me, but I decided to give it a try for a time. It didn't work. After all, whenever I did any type of lower body workout, I'd have pain in the lower part of my back. And sitting down, especially in a car, was very painful. Even small activities could cause my back to flare up. If I pushed with one leg on the assist of a bench press machine, I'd have to take a week off of work. Here was one more physical therapist that was not going to help me.

It was an absolutely brutal year for me. I didn't know what was wrong with me. I didn't know what to do next. Not one person I sought help from actually provided me with a solution to my pain. The pain was taking over my life—so much so that the topic of back pain was in almost every conversation I had with people. It became incredibly tiring just talking about it. At a certain point, I started lying so that I didn't have to talk about it anymore. I was so desperate for relief that I had put together a document detailing all of the people that I had seen. I was hoping that I could take this document to someone and they would fix me. My quality of life was hovering about as low as it could get at about a 1.

Year Two

In January, I saw another physical therapist. I saw her at seven in the morning for a one-hour therapy session before I went to work. Most of the exercises she gave me were very easy; none of them gave me any pain relief. I couldn't understand how any of it was going to help me. It felt like a joke. I'd lie there in pain, doing exercises that made no sense to me. One of the exercises was a crunch, a baby crunch, really, that required almost no effort.

I thought, *So let me see if I understand this. You are telling me that someone who was in absolute peak physical shape less than nine months ago now has a weak core and that is the cause of his pain? These baby exercises are going to relieve my pain?*

It was a joke. I went to the therapist three times a week for a month. Once I completed the recommended number of visits, I stopped going to see her. I wasn't getting any benefit from it.

Then one of my doctors recommended that I go see a pain medicine specialist who does injections into the spine. The injections usually consist of steroids and anti-inflammatory agents. There are many different types of injections. Their protocol called for a series of injections into my epidural space around the spinal cord, similar to what women in labor receive. The problem with these injections is that the doctors use a fluoroscope—basically an X-Ray machine that gives a continuous live picture—to guide them where to place the injection. Regardless of the high dose of radiation, it would be worth if it were to give me any pain relief.

On my first visit, the doctor tried to inject me through my sacrum. As you can imagine, the pain was almost unbearable. Finally, he gave up and did the injection in a different location. I barely made it through one injection—the pain was so bad. I had never dealt with such extremely intense pain like that before. If the first injection was that painful, I couldn't see how I was going to have any more. But I had to go through the process to see if it could help reduce the pain I was in. I didn't notice any improvement from the first injection. Luckily, the remaining injections were not as painful as the first one. After five injections, I still didn't get any relief.

One of the doctors had given me a book on how to treat your own back pain. The book told the story of a guy who went to see a doctor for his chronic back pain. The doctor told the patient to lie down on the table in the examination room until he returned. When the doctor finally got back, he was shocked by what he saw. The table had been left with one end higher than the other, and the patient had positioned himself on his stomach, with his head at the top, and his back extended severely backward.

The doctor was horrified. From what he knew about backs, it seemed like a terrible position for the patient to be in. But it actually helped relieve the patient's back pain.

The theory of the book was that people hurt their spine while bending forward, which causes bulges in the discs, which causes pain. If, instead of bending forward, a person bends backward, they can reduce the bulges and therefore reduce their pain. I tried to do these extension exercises religiously but it provided no relief. It was one more failed attempt to relieve my pain.

The doctors decided that, if the epidural injections provided no relief, then maybe other injections, like nerve root blocks, might be the answer. So, instead of injecting something into my spinal canal directly, they would inject where the nerves exited my spinal canal. So I started seeing another doctor who did injections in this way. As before, the process involved a series of injections. After the first injection, I was told that I should have immediate pain relief and that it would last for a certain amount of time. They asked me to walk up and down the stairs to see if I could sense any relief. I didn't.

On my way home, I stopped at a school and tried to lightly jog around the track to see if I would experience any sort of relief. I wanted so much for it to be the answer, but it didn't help. After all of the injections I had received, there was no significant reduction in my pain.

The doctor recommended that I get a discogram, a procedure that is used to pressurize the discs to try and recreate the pain. During the procedure, I was supposed to tell them how one pain compares to another. If they could duplicate the pain I usually feel, then they'd determine that my spinal discs were the likely cause of my pain. They decided to test the lower two discs of my spine because of the degenerative changes they seemed to demonstrate. Then, while I was lightly sedated, the doctor inserted a device into the disc to pressurize it. I have to tell you, I've been in pain before, but this was the most painful procedure I had ever had done in my life. The pain was so intense that I couldn't compare it to anything I have ever experienced. To give you an idea of what I went through, imagine getting stung by a bee. Then imagine having gasoline poured on your arm and setting it on fire. Now answer the following question: Does the pain in your arm feel like the bee sting pain?

The pain they created was so much more intense than my usual already-excruciating back pain that I couldn't give any definitive answers to their questions. So the test result was negative. Yet the determination they handed me was that one of my discs was holding pressure and the other one was not. I remember seeing a different doctor later and he wanted to redo the test. I told him there was no way in hell I would ever do that test again.

After all the injections and tests, I still had no significant improvement in my pain. I was living on muscle relaxants and just trying to make it through each day. I had gone to the very best back pain specialists in the Denver area searching for a solution. But I never found it.

By the fall of that year, I was so miserable that I was ready to try anything that might help. The cost didn't matter. I saw an article in the newspaper about a non-surgical alternative to back pain—a traction table. The theory was that by pulling on my spine, the pressure on my nerves from my discs would be relieved and give me some relief. I went for it. I paid $3700 (it was not covered by insurance) and went to lie on the traction table numerous times. It was the worst waste of money that I spent on my back pain so far and of course it gave me absolutely no relief.

I was in tremendous pain that year. If something fell on the floor, I would not pick it up. I was riddled with horrible guilt. I kept asking myself why I had played that stupid game again. I had hurt myself once and I should have known not to do it again, I thought. It replayed over and over in my head. But thankfully, I also discovered that I don't have an addictive personality. With all that pain, I could have easily become a raging alcoholic or a drug addict. But I had a job where I had to think for a living, and every time I tried a new pain medication, I could no longer think. Everything just became foggy. I'd rather live in pain than be a vegetable. My quality of life was about a 1 for the whole year.

Year Three

I started to feel like a guinea pig. I was willing to do any procedure that was requested of me with the hope of achieving some pain relief. Each time I went to a new doctor, I'd have to try to explain what had been done to me so far but because my history was so extensive, it was hard to explain it all.

A new doctor wanted to do injections into my facet joints. Maybe that's what was causing my pain. And of course, he needed a new MRI. He was located in Aurora, an hour's drive from where I worked in Longmont. I was living in Broomfield, which was a half an hour from work. The point is, I could barely sit down at all and yet I was driving for hours in search of relief. I went through another round of injections over the next six months. Not surprisingly, there was no improvement.

To make matters worse, I stubbed my toe getting out of bed, so I had a new pain in my toe in addition to my back pain. The pain in my toe got so bad that I had to see a doctor for it. I started with X-Rays, an MRI, and injections. I never seemed to get any relief. I could barely sit in my car to begin with and now my foot hurt so bad that I could barely drive. One Saturday, I was out driving, and when I returned home and pulled into my driveway, I simply broke down. I just couldn't deal with all of it anymore.

Why was no one helping me? Day after day, the pain was wearing on me. I think it was the first time that it started to sink in that maybe there really wasn't a way out of my pain. I was starting to have some very dark thoughts and it scared the hell out of me.

The doctor recommended foot surgery, so I decided to have it. After the surgery, I needed physical therapy on my foot. When I'd see the therapist, she'd work on my toe, usually causing extreme pain. But one day the therapist moved my toe and the pain in my toe disappeared. I was thrilled. Finally, I had some relief. *Now*, I thought, *I can try to fix my back again.*

I got a referral from my doctor for physical therapy for my back and I continued to get work done with the same therapist. I continued there for a full year. But unfortunately, it was a complete failure.

In addition to getting physical therapy, I got bounced around to different pain medicine specialists. I started seeing someone else in Denver who told me that they did their injections differently than the others. They told me that they'd inject in a different spot or with a different solution and I should get some result from it. Of course, I would need to do a whole series of injections to have any hope of improvement. Sometimes it seemed to feel a little better but maybe it was just hope masking the pain. In the end, I got no pain relief.

One of my pain medicine specialists recommended I try a new procedure. Since the results of the discogram suggested that one of my discs was not holding pressure, that disc might be the cause of my pain. So he wanted to do a procedure that would place a wire around the inside of my disc that would then be heated to a high temperature. The goal was to seal up the cracks in my disc and possibly shrink my disc to reduce any nerve irritation. It didn't work. The worst part was that this doctor was located in Fort Collins, which was at least 45 minutes from work, in the opposite direction of where I lived. Adding insult to injury, the doctor would always triple book his patients. It would take at least two hours just to get into see him.

In December, my company took all of the employees in my department out for lunch to celebrate the holidays. The company had merged with another company and we were hearing there would be massive layoffs. Let's just say the mood for the lunch was not very jovial. My pain was so bad that I didn't think I could even make it through lunch. Sitting down was almost impossible.

Within a couple of weeks, I found out I had been laid off. Now it may not sound like a good thing, but at least I didn't have to sit all day in terrible pain. Just to not have to sit in my car made my life somewhat bearable. My quality of life had increased to a 2 because I stopped working. Maybe with a little more time, my pain would calm down and I could go back to work. I had planned to spend the Christmas holiday with my parents but they lived five hours away by car. No way could I make the drive. Thankfully, a friend of mine from my hometown happened to be driving back to our old stomping grounds, so he gave me a ride. If not for him, I would have celebrated Christmas at home, alone.

Year Four

I started the year off with a lot of back pain and no job. And the clock was ticking: my insurance was going to run out as soon as my severance package was up and that would spell the end of my healthcare. I saw a new physical therapist during the first two months of the year while I continued searching for an orthopedic surgeon who might be able to help me. Someone recommended a surgeon in Boulder, so I made an appointment to see him. It took two weeks to get in to see him. I brought all of my records with me and hoped and prayed that the new doc had some tricks up his sleeve that all the others didn't have. I kept thinking that there had to be something that was missing that would just magically cure me. But it wasn't so with this doctor.

Since I was unemployed and needed an income, I purchased an investment property near my parents' home. The problem was, the property was five hours away and it needed some work. So I had to drive there, a trip that was excruciating for me. I would manage until my pain level was off the charts and then I'd get out of the car. My right leg would go numb and my pelvis would feel like it was on fire. I couldn't go more than 30 minutes before the pain was unbearable. I couldn't do any of the physical work myself anyway. If I moved the wrong way, the pain level would skyrocket. Luckily, I was offered a job and I was able to hire out the remaining work.

Since I needed the medical benefits, I started the new job immediately, but the pain became unbearable almost immediately. Once again, I was stuck sitting on the job all day long. Plus, I'd have to sit in the car to drive there and back. With the stress that came with a new job, things became overwhelming for me. My quality of life fell back to a 1.

I was dreading the day they asked me to travel.

At least I had medical benefits. I went back to the pain medicine specialist and started doing more injections. Because I was getting no relief at all, I spent numerous hours traveling to new doctors. One doctor would recommend a consultation with another doctor. Each time I saw a new practitioner I needed to get an updated MRI. At that point, I had so much pain all over my body that it was hard to figure out what the issue really was.

I had gone back to one of my orthopedic surgeons. It was interesting because he had previously told me that there was nothing that he could do for me. But when I went back to see him, a bulge in a disc magically appeared in the MRI that he could now operate on. It was a miracle. The bulge may be responsible for all of my pain, I was told.

It was the first time since I started seeking help for my pain that anyone had offered a surgical option. Since I felt I had no choice, I decided to go ahead with it. The procedure, a microdiscectomy, entails cutting out the small portion of the disc that may be impinging on the nerves. It only required a small incision and was an outpatient procedure. Well, if that was the procedure that was going to change my life, I was sadly disappointed. There was no change in my health.

Now what? It was just one sad miserable day after another.

One morning, I woke up and, for a moment, I was pain-free. I thought maybe it was all just a bad dream. Then I felt the pain creep back in. I heard that our muscles are paralyzed when we sleep and they come to life as we wake up. I do not know if it's true or not but that's what it felt like. I really didn't even want to get out of bed.

At that point, I was feeling very low. My quality of life was about 0.5 again. I just couldn't do it anymore. I had seen numerous doctors, surgeons, pain medicine specialists, and physical therapists and not one of them had ever provided me with a solution for my debilitating chronic back pain. No one knew what was wrong with me. I couldn't even make it through one day without pain. I couldn't do any physical activity that I once loved to do. My mountain bike and tennis racquets were gathering dust. Every day was a struggle.

I could hardly find any reason to continue living. I started to think of ways that I could kill myself. Suicide seemed like my only option. I tried to find anything that would give me a reason to hang on. Luckily I didn't have a gun in my house or it may have been all over for me. I just didn't know what to do. I just kept living one sad miserable day at a time. Even though my work was stressful, and making it through the day was unbearable, work actually provided a certain amount of distraction from the pain. If I had been home alone all day it might have been the end of me.

I went to a follow up appointment with a pain medicine specialist. He took one look at me and could tell I was not doing well. I saw the panic in his face. He immediately prescribed a cocktail of pain medicine and anti-depressants and told me the story of another patient that they couldn't get a hold of. He never said it, but I assumed that the patient killed himself because of the pain. I think he was trying to scare me into taking the medications. I think he thought that I might be next.

The only good thing that came out of that office visit was that I learned about artificial discs. I was being told repeatedly that my discs were the cause of my pain. If I were to replace my discs, I thought, then maybe I could stop the horrible pain I was feeling. He referred me to a doctor who was performing clinical trials with artificial discs in Denver. What are the odds that the top specialist for artificial discs was a few miles away from my house? I had always believed that there was some surgery out there that would fix me. This was cutting-edge new technology. Things were looking up.

I started doing as much research as I could do on artificial discs. They were not approved in the U.S., but they were being done overseas. I was lucky enough to have enough equity in my house that, worst-case scenario, I could sell my house, fly to Europe, and pay for the procedure out of pocket. It was my only hope and it was the only thing that got me through the rest of year. Just the thought that I might get artificial discs increased my quality of life to a 2.

Year Five

The moment I had been dreading since I started my new job had finally come to pass. My company asked me to travel to Japan for two weeks. Once again, I was scared to death. Once again, I felt like I would lose my job if I didn't go.

I used my airline miles and upgraded to business class so I could lie down, which made the trip a little easier. I arrived in

Tokyo at 4 p.m. and sat on a bus for four hours to get to my hotel due to the traffic. I somehow managed to get there without wanting to put a bullet in my head. Just being in a foreign country halfway around the world was stressful enough, but having intense pain in my back on top of it made it unbearable. So I counted the days until it was all over. I had done what was asked of me and I figured I might be able to keep my job a little longer because of it. I was able to endure the plane ride home thanks to business class. My QOL was a 1 for the trip. My stress level slowly came down as I thought about continuing my quest to fix my back.

I finally felt hopeful. I started to believe that my new doctor was the one person that could take my pain away. I explained my rather extensive medical history to him. He told me he was conducting randomized blind clinical trial on a new artificial disc. Going into the procedure, each patient wouldn't know if they were getting artificial discs or a fusion procedure. He told me that, for every patient, two would get an artificial disc and one would get a fusion. It wasn't until the patient woke up that they would learn which procedure they had received.

But there was good news and bad news. The bad news was that the clinical trial was over; they were not accepting any more patients. The good news was that they were still going to allow people to receive the artificial discs only. This was part of the study—just not randomized blind. I was horrified with the prospect of a fusion, so to be able to receive artificial discs, in the U.S., and have insurance pay for it was really great news. The doctor had decided that I needed to have two levels replaced—I would have two new discs. I would be one of the first people ever to have two levels of artificial discs. I was incredibly excited.

Because it was such an extensive surgery, I needed to undergo a multitude of tests before the procedure could happen. Of course, I needed a new MRI, also. The list of risks was incredible. I was so broken that I felt I had no choice but to do the surgery. Some of the doctors even commented that I was way too young to be undergoing the new surgery.

The procedure required that the doctors go through my stomach to replace my discs. There would be two surgeons: one who would open me up and the other would replace my discs. My original discs would be removed and grooves would be cut into my vertebrae to receive the artificial discs. These artificial discs were two pieces of metal with a keel on the back and a plastic insert in the middle. A ball and socket design. Apparently new bone would grow around the keel and seal it in place.

The surgery was in late August. With all the preamble, I had waited almost a year for the procedure. I was very excited because I believed it was going to be the procedure that would finally give me my life back.

In the hospital after the procedure, I couldn't sleep through the night because I got woken up every hour to make sure that I was alive. After two nights in the hospital, I told them I was going home. The nurses look at me in disbelief. Once they removed the catheter, I popped a couple of painkillers and walked out the door.

After a couple more days, I started walking around the park. In a little over a week, I went back to work. I had been living in so much pain that dealing with the surgical pain on top of my normal pain didn't change things much.

Going through such an extensive procedure was brutal on my system. I was hoping for a silver lining—that it would have been worth all the pain and suffering. I kept expecting that with time I would be in less and less pain. But as the surgical pain slowly dissipated, I could still feel the same old back pain. Nothing seemed to be different. I went back to the physical therapist that I was seeing before the surgery, hoping it would help speed up the improvement. Even with everything I had been through, my quality of life was holding at a 1.

Year Six

My physical therapist suggested that I work with a massage therapist. My muscles were terribly tight and she thought that some massage might help as well as kick-start the physical therapy process, too. She was right; my muscles were so tight that I pulled my left hamstring just stepping onto an elliptical machine. I'd get a massage every Saturday and get physical therapy during the week. The therapist said massaging my muscles was like massaging a piece of steel. Occasionally, I'd get a little temporary relief from the massage, but it didn't last very long. By the time I saw her again the following week; it was like starting all over again, massaging the same piece of steel. I wasn't making any headway, and it was costing me a lot of money. I had to pay for the massage out of pocket since it wasn't covered by my insurance.

Because I was part of a clinical trial, I had to have regular follow-up visits with the surgeon. I'd get X-Rays and a quick office visit, which included simple movement tests. It was clear that my muscles were all locked up. I had been hurt for so long that I was constantly in protective mode. The doctor told me that I needed to start moving. He told me to start with simple things like bending down and touching my toes or bending side to side. Believe it or not, it was incredibly hard for me to do those things. I was scared to death just to bend forward; after all, it could easily cause a bout of pain that would last a year. But the goal of the medical team was to get me to try to start doing things that I enjoyed, like golf or tennis. Slowly, I tried to coax my body into letting me do some of those things, but it was not happy. To swing a golf club seemed like an impossible task.

I did notice one interesting thing on my X-Rays: it looked like my pelvis was tilted to one side. It seemed obvious to me that there was some sort of alignment issue going on: the discs seemed to be tilted to compensate for the small pelvic shift. When I asked the surgeon about it, all he said was not to worry about it. What was important was that the discs were in alignment, he said.

Along with the usual pain in my back, I started to experience intense pain in my right leg, too. My surgeon concluded that I had nerve damage so he recommended that I see a neurologist. My nerves were probably overstretched when I had the disc replacement surgery. The neurologist told me that nerves grow about 1mm per month and that I would heal. It was just going to take some time.

By late spring, it was very hard for me to continue working at my job day after day. The trauma of the surgery, along with the continual pain and stress I had from work, was getting to be too much for me. My body was seizing up and sitting at a desk all day was not helping either. I realized I needed to take some time off of work. I got the doctor to sign off on a disability leave and I took most of the summer off.

I don't know how it happened, but I was able to continue to go to physical therapy sessions even though I had exceeded the number of visits I was granted. So throughout the summer I continued to get physical therapy. The therapist had me wear a sacroiliac belt, a belt that's worn around the lower part of the pelvis to help keep the sacrum in alignment. The therapist noticed that my pelvis was tilted abnormally.

We developed a routine. I'd be in unbearable pain and go see her for some soft tissue work. From that, my body would calm down slightly. In a couple days, the pain would get unbearable again, and I'd go in to see her again. It became obvious to me that she had absolutely no idea what was wrong with me. But, as long as the insurance was paying for it, she would continue to see me. It didn't matter to her if I improved or not. At no time was there any significant reduction in my pain.

For almost nine months, I got physical therapy and it did absolutely nothing for me. It also became obvious to me that the disc replacement surgery had been a complete failure.

When I look back at that surgery, I find it interesting that every one of my tests came back negative. The discogram came back negative; no one could successfully argue that my discs were the cause of my pain. Yet they told me I was still considered a good candidate for the procedure. No wonder I failed the surgery.

The one thing that I have learned is that when you are in enough pain, someone will operate. The outcome does not matter.

When summer was over, I went back to work. I was still living with agonizing pain, but the time off from work helped my mood a little. Then I found out that even though the doctor had signed off on the disability application, the insurance company denied my claim. I received no money for the time off. Seemed to be just the way my luck was running. Because I was back at work, my quality of life was back at a 1. What a horrible life I was living.

Year Seven

Even though it seemed completely useless, I continued to go to physical therapy and I was still paying out of pocket to get my steel-like muscles massaged. The follow-up appointments I had with the surgeon just led me to see more doctors who had no answers. My pain was crippling me and I started taking anti-seizure medication. I was also given an electrical stimulation device that I was told to use on my own to relax my tight muscles. It didn't help.

Someone had pointed me in the direction of an alternative medicine doctor in Boulder. He didn't accept any insurance, but I had heard good things about him. He did an examination and concluded that I had a leg length discrepancy. My right leg was shorter than my left. Then he showed me that my orthotics were wrong. There was more lift on the left side than the right and this was causing an even shorter right leg. He wanted me to get an X-Ray at a hospital where he had setup a plumb bob that would show me how far off my pelvis was. He recommended that I replace my orthotics or stop wearing them. I was already on my third pair since I hurt my back. He also recommended that I wear a heel lift in my right shoe. I couldn't figure out what he was showing me and I was not sure if this was the cause of my pain. I stopped wearing my orthotics and started wearing the heel lift. I kept expecting some great improvement in my health but it never came. I abandoned his plan fairly quickly.

The company that I was working for was a startup and we had the sense that it wasn't going to succeed. The latest product that we were developing had to be finished on time so a team of employees would be sent to the factory in China for one month. I was dreading having to travel again but I had no choice; I had to go. I was able to get through the Japan trip, barely, so I thought I could survive it. But I would not travel without a business class ticket. That would help me get through the first leg of the trip—getting there.

Once there, we worked very long days. It was brutal for a healthy person; for me, it was unbearable. The combination of long days and the 12-hour time difference sent me into a dark hole. I hit rock bottom. I was ready to quit my job, get on a plane, and fly home. My quality of life was a 0.5 again.

My boss asked me if I could stay one more week and I told him there was absolutely no way. My mood improved the moment I walked on to the plane. No matter how hard this flight might be on me, I was going home. Once home, I set out again to fix my back.

I heard about a physical therapist in Denver who was said to be one of the best in his field. When I went to see him, he did an examination and told me there was nothing wrong with me. I was told to start doing squats and some other exercises and I would be fine. So I went to the gym, tried the exercises, and wound up in horrible pain. I couldn't do what he asked. He was of no benefit to me.

It was at this point that I had to come to the clear realization that this was as good as my life was ever going to get. I was going to live the rest of my life in pain. I could either do these activities with a lot of pain or I could sit on the couch. My only solution was to grin and bear it. I would play a few holes of golf until my right leg would go numb. And I would stop once the pain became excruciating.

For the first time in a long time, I got on my mountain bike to attempt a ride. I was almost done with the ride when I hit a rock that was covered with leaves. One of my hands slipped off the handlebars and my head jolted forward. When I got off the bike, I noticed some pain in my neck.

The neck pain got worse and worse and eventually became just as severe as the pain in my back. Now I had to deal with neck pain along with my back pain. How much worse could my life get?

I had to seek treatment immediately. There was a pain medicine specialist with an office near my house so I went to see him for weekly injections. He treated both my back and my neck and told me that my sacrum was fused together on the left side. Was this the cause of my pain? He recommended I try acupuncture with him. It did me no good whatsoever.

In December, the company that I was working for went out of business. I was out of a job one more time. Once my severance was up, I would have no more health insurance again. What a good way to end the year. My quality of life was on fumes at 1.5.

Year Eight

I started out the New Year knowing that I would only have health insurance for three more months. I continued the treatment path that I was on. I did more injections in my neck and the back; I continued with the physical therapy.

Then one day, my insurance ran out. My physical therapist was more than happy to continue to see me at $55 per visit and, if it actually offered any light at the end of the tunnel, I would have continued with her. But it all seemed so useless to me. I stopped all treatment.

The amount of pain I was experiencing was barely manageable so I hardly did anything else but sit on the couch all day. Sometimes I'd go to the gym and try to do the exercises that the physical therapist gave me but it only caused more pain. Over time, the pain eventually calmed down a little so I tried to resume more activities. But in the end, the result was always the same: more pain.

I found out that a lot of the employees from the company I had worked for had moved to Southern California. A disk drive company in Lake Forest was hiring and they offered me a job. I was very ready to leave cold Colorado—I just wasn't sure I could handle sitting at a desk all day. If they had asked me to do any physical work or travel, I wouldn't even have considered taking the job. If they said the job is yours but you have to drive out here, I would have turned it down. There was no way I would have even passed a physical. But I figured I should take the job; worst-case scenario, I could go on disability if I needed to.

When I started at the new company, my pain immediately got worse just from sitting all day. I found a doctor right away. Of course, he needed me to get a new MRI. But my artificial discs had made my MRI unreadable, so, no more MRIs. The doctor was my primary care physician. I knew he would be of no help to me but he might possibly know someone who might be able to help. Because he had a chiropractor in his office, he recommended me to him. I was very hesitant because I had seen chiropractors in the past and had experienced no improvement from their work on me. But I went ahead. The treatment plan called for multiple visits per week for four to six weeks.

Then something absolutely amazing happened. For the first time, something was reducing my pain. This chiropractor was actually helping me. I couldn't believe it.

The only problem was that the pain relief was temporary. If I made the wrong movement, I would be right back where I started, in pain again. Thus began my chiropractic dependency. I would have an adjustment and hope that it would hold as long as possible. I would bend or twist and there goes the adjustment. Even the smallest of movements would bring me back out of alignment. I would grab the groceries out of my car and I would come out of alignment.

I needed about two adjustments per week. He was adjusting both my back and neck at the same time. Even though I was stuck in this repetitive cycle with the chiropractor, my life had improved. My body would be a little inflamed after each adjustment but my pain would significantly decrease.

I couldn't believe it. I had actually found something that was helping me to be more active. I'd ride my bike until I was out of alignment and then go to the chiropractor. I'd play golf until I was out of alignment and then go to the chiropractor. The only problem was that when I would come out of alignment, the pain was very hard to deal with. If I was playing golf and got out of alignment by the third hole, the rest of the round was absolutely miserable for me. My right leg would go numb and my lower back would ache. I'd never do any warm-ups because I didn't want to pull anything out before even getting started. It was my life. If I had given it to someone else they would have said they were completely disabled. I just lived with it because it was all I could do.

Since I was starting to learn how my alignment was responsible for my pain, I thought I would try going back to a physical therapist. I thought physical therapy might work now that I was in alignment. I explained to the therapist how the chiropractor had treated me and his response was to show me a method to adjust my own back. It made some sense to me, so I stopped seeing the chiropractor for a short time.

But I tried the alignment technique for a while and ended up back in miserable pain. It was obvious that the physical therapist had no idea what the chiropractor did. His treatment method didn't work. It absolutely ruined my Christmas because I was in severe pain. I went back to the chiropractor and immediately felt better.

Somehow I had developed an inguinal hernia that was causing me some discomfort. I couldn't believe that I had one more thing to deal with in my life. But because I had learned about chiropractic care, I was doing much better and started feeling a little hopeful. If I acted like a robot and avoided activity, I'd be able to have several days with significantly less pain. My mood was definitely better and my quality of life rose to a 4.

Chapter 2
The Second Eight Years

Year Nine

The chiropractor became my ongoing, continuous resource for pain relief. I saw him at least twice a week and when my insurance ran out, I paid $65 out of pocket to be able to keep seeing him. But it wasn't enough: I spent more time out of alignment than in alignment. If I got out of alignment on a Friday evening, I'd spend the entire weekend on the couch in excruciating pain. It wouldn't be until after my morning meetings at work that I'd be able to get in to see the chiropractor and straighten myself out.

This chiropractor told me there was nothing that could be done to fix me. He said, "Just go have fun and come in to see me when you need it." So I saw him a lot. Most visits only took five or ten minutes max. I only needed a simple adjustment. He'd almost always produce a pop that would confirm that the adjustment was complete.

I even tried to see if I could adjust my back by myself. I placed weights on my legs and rotated my torso. I could sometimes create a pop but I could never quite get the adjustment right. And that was just my back. My neck was in so much pain that I could only look up or down for a few minutes. I'd have to have the chiropractor adjust it every time I went in to see him.

When it came to sports and activities like golf, it was hit or miss. I knew that anything like that would make me feel worse but I tried to get in a little fun if I could. If my pain level was already pretty high, then I wouldn't even attempt it. But if I thought I could get in a little activity without too much trouble, I'd go for it.

I had to pay attention to what did and what didn't cause problems with my back or neck. Swinging a golf club actually wasn't a problem since rotating my body to swing the club didn't cause much pain. But when I experienced any kind of sudden impact, even something as seemingly benign as sticking the club into the ground, my back would immediately get out of alignment and I'd be in pain. I'd have to be careful each time I went to pull my clubs out of my car for fear that it would put my back out of alignment. Bending over and lifting things was asking for trouble. Even simple tasks like opening a jar with a tight lid was very hard for me and would cause pain.

My quality of life was at a 3 that year.

Year Ten

After dealing with my hernia for over a year, I decided to take care of it. I had the procedure done on a Friday so I'd have the weekend to recover. When I went home on Friday, the pain wasn't so bad so I decided not to fill my prescription for pain medicine. It was a huge mistake. By Saturday, the pain was so intense that I just had to lie in bed without moving a muscle. I remember thinking that if I ever wanted to torture someone, this would be a great way to do it. By Monday the pain had calmed down and I was back at work. I told the doctor that I did not take any pain medication and he said I was the only patient he's ever known who didn't take it. I think I made it through because I was used to living with a very high pain threshold.

As soon as the pain from the hernia surgery reduced a little, I went back into my chiropractic cycle. I saw my primary chiropractor a few times a week and saw other chiropractors when my guy was not around or when I traveled. I paid for them out of pocket.

I couldn't maintain my alignment at all. All week, I'd work, come home, take off my shoes, sit down on my couch, and get out of alignment. The weekend was a loss. My muscles were so tight that I ached all over. When I tried to simply stretch my calves, I'd go out of alignment.

One of the doors to the office building at work had gotten so hard for me to open that I couldn't open it without pulling my back out. So I'd walk around to the other side of the building and go in that way instead. If I was feeling reasonably good, I'd ride my bike at lunch. But once I was on the bike, if I wanted to look behind me, I could only look over one shoulder. Choosing the wrong side would cause my back to go out. When I'd walk, I avoided sidewalks because the inevitable slope of the driveways I'd have to cross exacerbated my back and put me in pain. The street, on the other hand, was predictably flat and back-friendly.

I could always tell when my back was out of alignment because that's when the pain was at its worst. I decided to try physical therapy again, but I came to realize that my physical therapist didn't have a clue about whether or not I was in alignment. Every time I walked into her office, I'd tell her that I was out of alignment, and she'd look at me and say, "No you're not." So I'd walk out her office, go back to my chiropractor for an adjustment, and get the pain relief I was hoping for. I realized that there's a huge disconnect between what chiropractors do and what physical therapists do. The physical therapist didn't understand what the chiropractor did. I also came to understand that it was useless to do the physical therapy if my back was out of alignment because my nervous system was constantly being irritated.

Someone told me about a procedure called *prolotherapy*. It consists of a series of injections that were different from the other injections that I had gotten. Instead of injecting steroids near the nerves, the prolotherapist injects an irritant into the ligaments, which would cause inflammation to occur and the inflammation would trigger the ligaments to repair themselves. When I went in to find out about it for myself, I was told that the loose ligaments were likely to be the cause of my pain. Even though the procedure wasn't covered by my insurance, I was so desperate that I decided to try it.

Year Eleven

I got prolotherapy injections about once a month for six months and, for some reason, I kept expecting that my health would get better. I paid $1900 for the privilege, but it didn't really give me any pain relief. It was just another failed procedure and another huge waste of money.

My health and the level of pain I experienced would vary every day. A friend of mine came to visit me and we played golf at a small Par 3 course. That was about all I was willing to try. I played a few holes and then made one wrong move and the pain was back in full force. My friend noticed that I could barely swing a club. He definitely noticed a change in my game.

A few months later, he came back out to visit with his family. They had a multiday pass at Disneyland, so one day I went with them to join in the fun. I told them that I absolutely couldn't get on any rides. They might seem like nothing to everyone else but they were catastrophic to me. Thankfully, I made it through the day and didn't pull my back out.

Later in the week, I took a day off from work to hang out with my friend and his family. We played some tennis in the morning and by some miracle I was relatively pain free. They had one last day at Disneyland and my friend talked me into going on one ride. I reluctantly agreed.

I chose a ride that did not look bad from the ground. I figured that, worst-case scenario, it would just pull my back out and I'd just go see the chiropractor again afterwards. Not surprisingly, we waited in line forever until it was finally our turn. I was scared to death; I knew it was a bad idea. When the ride was over, it took a minute for the shock to wear off. Slowly, the pain got worse and worse. It had definitely pulled my back out. In minutes, I was miserable and I just walked around in disbelief. I walked out of the park, hopped into a taxi, and went home. The rest of the day was a catastrophe.

I went to see my chiropractor as soon as I could the next day. He told me that my back was significantly out of alignment and I wasn't surprised. The pain didn't calm down right away like it normally did after an adjustment. I barely made it through the day and the rest of the weekend was absolutely brutal. I started to think that I couldn't go on like this.

Somehow on Monday I went back to work. If I was barely hanging on before, I wasn't anymore. Every day was one agonizing day after another. It took all I had to just make it through the day. The neurological pain was debilitating. My quality of life plummeted to a 0.5.

I went to see a pain medicine specialist to see if I could go on disability leave. The doctor wanted to see if any medications could help me and he wanted to try some injections before he would be willing to sign off on the disability paperwork. He gave me drugs to try but they were intolerable to me; they all just put me into a vegetative state. He gave me multiple injections with no success. Then he did a nerve conduction test and found nerve damage in both legs. He signed the disability papers and that was it.

I had a job that paid over $100,000 a year. It required no physical work, no travel, and still I couldn't do it. Just sitting at a desk was an impossibly hard task for me. I had no choice but to walk away; I just couldn't continue with all the pain anymore. My quality of life had been so poor for so long that even I was surprised I had made it this far. I couldn't even remember the last time I had been pain free because it has been so long.

I never felt quite at home in California and it was way too expensive to live there, so I decided to move to Las Vegas. I had enough money to sustain me for a while. I made a new plan: I'd live there until my money ran out and then I'd take my own life. Clearly, there was no one who could help me, so I figured I'd just try to enjoy what was left.

I did not know anyone in Las Vegas, but it wasn't cold there and I liked to play poker. So it seemed like a good choice. Since sitting was almost impossible for me, you'd think that poker would be the last thing I'd want to do. But there was hardly anything I could do anyway, so I enjoyed myself. I'd sit there until I couldn't take the pain anymore, then I'd stand up. If someone bumped into the back of my chair, my back would go out of alignment and I'd be in terrible pain.

I was having severe issues with my right foot. Any slight temperature difference and my foot would ache terribly. I'd wear socks in bed because if I pulled my foot out of the covers and the air conditioner blew on it, it would hurt. My right leg was really cold. It was determined that I had drop foot so I started wearing a device that would support my foot. I was also taking nerve support supplements.

I found chiropractors in the area who would help me function. I started getting regular massages again, too, because my muscles were all locked up. Unfortunately, the massage was completely useless; the therapist could never make any headway. One therapist actually told me that I should stop seeing her because I was just wasting my money. I was shocked. She was the only person I had ever met in healthcare who was truly honest. Everyone else I had sought for treatment would have continued to see me regardless of the outcome.

Year Twelve

I had a follow-up appointment with a pain medicine specialist I had seen in California and I had to drive there. It is less than a five-hour trip but even five minutes in the car was still extremely rough for me to endure. The drive was insufferable but I made it and had my appointment with the doctor. My friend invited me to dinner so I planned to stay the night at his house and then drive home the next day. After dinner, I took a hot bath and went to bed, but I was in too much pain to sleep. I lay there as long as I could, but at about 4 a.m., I got up and left for the long drive home. I drove for as long as I could until the pain got too unbearable, and then I'd stop and get out. I stopped a million times. I realized I could never do a trip like that again. Note to self: No more road trips in my future.

My manager called me and told me that I was being laid off. I was given a severance package and three months' of health insurance.

I decided to see a physical therapist. She told me that I needed a heel lift in my shoe and then proceeded to sell me several of them. Then she recommended that I see somebody else who showed me some stretches to do. She demonstrated the movements to me but she wouldn't provide me with a hard copy of the exercises to take home. I thought, *This is part of physical therapy now?* I tried to do her exercises along with the regular physical therapy and got nothing out of it.

Only chiropractic treatments provided me with any kind of relief from my back and neck pain. A friend recommended another chiropractor to me. For $50 a visit, he was sure he could really help me, he said. It would only take 12 visits and I'd feel like a new person, he told me. Everyone I see seems to have some grand plan that will make your life so much better. However, after their course of treatments fails, they have no problem continuing to treat you even though there is no major improvement. Why does it seem like used car salesmen are running our healthcare system? After his treatment ended, I went to the cheapest chiropractor that I could find. I could get the same temporary relief from someone who charges a lot less.

Someone recommended that I see a C.H.E.K. practitioner, something like a personal trainer. I was desperate for relief so I went to see her. She did what she called a "thorough examination" and was convinced that she could fix my body. She thought I had a gluten allergy and told me that I should go gluten-free. I told her that if she proves it, I'd do it. She was telling some allergy is causing my debilitating pain? Seemed like crap to me. I'd had so much smoke blown up my ass by that point that I could smell bullshit from a mile away. Her recommended course of treatment was almost identical to physical therapy.

Someone else pointed me in the direction of a medical massage therapist. Medical massage was supposed to be better than regular massage. *At $105 a visit, it better be*, I thought. But this therapist actually did me a favor: he actually showed me how my pelvis was misaligned. It had been pointed out to me before, but I couldn't figure out if that was the true cause of my pain. I tried wearing a heel lift again, but it gave me very little improvement in pain. This guy actually told me that if wearing the heel lift in one shoe didn't help then I should try it in the other shoe. That seemed absolutely insane to me! After several thousand dollars and not much relief, I stopped seeing him. I returned to a lower cost massage therapist once more.

The new massage therapist recommended that I see a fascial stretch therapist. A couple of visits couldn't hurt, I figured, so I went for it. The fascial stretch therapist physically moved parts of my body to help me regain movement in my joints and muscles. Believe it or not, I absolutely loved the therapy because my body was seized up and it needed to move. At the same time I loved it, I wasn't seeing an improvement in my condition. I seemed to be starting over every time I came for an appointment. So I discontinued treatment.

I went to see a local pain medicine specialist so I could continue with my disability leave. He wanted to implant an electrical stimulator in my back. I turned it down. I went to see a neurologist to see if he could help me. He wanted to do all of the usual tests and prescribe the usual drugs. I couldn't afford to do it out of pocket, so I did nothing. My quality of life was hovering at a 2.

Year Thirteen

The massage therapist recommended that I try to do some yoga along with the massage to help me loosen up my muscles more quickly. I had never done yoga before. Now I was doing hot yoga and it was intense. For a long time, I had been afraid to bend down and touch my toes and there I was, bending down and pulling. I was sure that it was going to break me, but it didn't. In fact, I started noticing a real change in my body. I was slowly starting to shift out of a tight, locked up condition; several muscles were even relaxing a little.

While the yoga improved my condition by helping me loosen up a bit, it did not help me with my stability issue. My condition was incredibly unstable because so many simple, normal movements would end up dislocating my spine. I had to be extremely careful, or else I'd have to go back to the chiropractor as soon as possible.

Year Fourteen

I took a trip to my parent's home and met a local chiropractor, George Evans. Like the medical massage therapist, George showed me how my pelvis was out of alignment. He also told me how a heel lift could put me back into alignment. He showed me how the misalignment was also causing my neck pain because my head was leaning to one side. So I started wearing a heel lift again. I could see a very small improvement but my condition still wasn't stabilizing. Almost any movement would pull my spine out of alignment.

Doing yoga fairly regularly helped ease my pain enough to try a trip to Hawaii, so off I went. Unfortunately, as soon as I got on the plane, things started going downhill and I realized it was a bad idea. When I arrived on the island, I sought out a chiropractor immediately. After working on me, he recommended that I get a massage because he thought the plane ride had been disastrous on my back. So I went to the massage therapist who felt compelled to tell me that there was nothing wrong with me other than muscle tightness. He said that I did not need the heel lift after all so I removed it.

I spent more time in pain and more money on my own healthcare than anything else I did on that trip. I just wanted to go home. And then I had to endure the miserable plane ride back.

Year Fifteen

The yoga was loosening me up a little but it could only get me so far. I needed more aggressive stretching and I needed someone who could help me get my muscles moving again. I decided to try fascial stretching again. It actually forced my body to move, and I saw improvement that I didn't get from yoga. Having someone stretch me was far more effective than doing it alone, but it wasn't helping me gain any ground in keeping my back from dislocating so quickly. After $2400 worth of treatments, I stopped getting the fascial work. It was obvious this fascial stretch therapist did not know how to fix my body.

I switched to a business chain of chiropractors who were charging much less than what I had been paying. They had several offices in the area, which made it easier for me to see them. The only challenge was to find a chiropractor who was actually competent. It took me a while to find the offices with the best chiropractors.

Year Sixteen

Again, the instability of my condition was making life very difficult for me. I had to be very careful to modify even the simplest tasks of life to avoid pulling my back out of alignment. It was making me crazy. When it came to opening the refrigerator, for example, instead of pulling on the door, I'd put my thumb on one door, and the fingers of the same hand on the other door, so that I'd only use the strength of my hand to get the door open. I'd be very careful driving over speed bumps. I could only take them head on otherwise the shifting of the car would pull me out of alignment. Just turning over in bed could pull my back out. If I needed to turn in bed, I'd put my legs straight and slowly roll over. If I wanted to shut off my nightstand light, I'd have to get out of bed, shut it off, and get back in bed slowly. If I reached the wrong way, my chiropractor made more money.

To avoid dislocating my spine, I had become like a robot, limiting my movements to reduce the risk to a minimum. My poor health had sent me to the land of misfit people: a very expensive place to live. I was one step away from ending it all. If I had gotten some fatal disease like cancer I'd have chosen to not fight it.

I became long-term unemployed. I had filed for disability but was denied it. Even though I had an extensive and debilitating health issue, it was determined that I could still work some job. I am not sure where such a job exists that would allow me to do no physical work, no prolonged sitting or standing, no bending, no lifting, no twisting, and no travel. Yet it would allow me to lie down if needed.

I could not recall one day in the last sixteenth years that I was free of pain. On my best day, my quality of life was a whopping 4. Because I had had so many miserable days, my average quality of life through all those years was maybe 1.5. Some people lead extraordinary lives. My life has been horrendously bad. I had spent over $75,000 out of my own pocket trying to treat my torturous back pain. It had affected every part of my life. I knew that I was going to take the pain to my grave.

Then one day, something changed. I went back to see George Evans, the chiropractor. He explained to me why the heel lift had been helping me and I started to understand that the position of my pelvis might actually be contributing to my chronic pain more than I had realized. He planted a seed in my mind that would soon germinate.

Chapter 3
Baby Steps

The figure on the right side shows how a healthy, normal body is supposed to look. Everything is in alignment. The pelvis is level, the shoulders are level, and the head is straight.

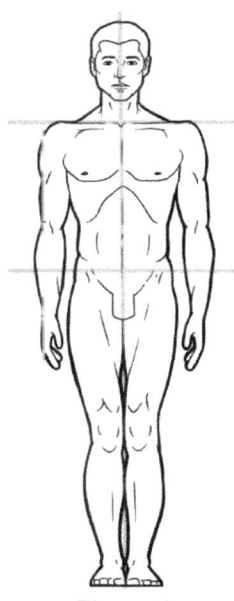

Figure 1

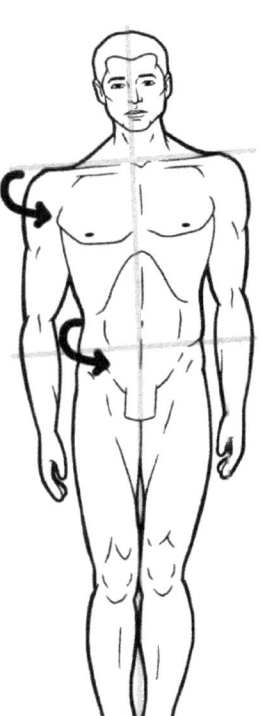

Figure 2

But this was how my body was lined up. After years of back pain, my body was really crooked.

My body was leaning to the right. My pelvis was higher on the left side than the right. My belly button was shifted to the left. My left shoulder was higher than my right and my head was tilted to the right and rotated to the left.

This was what George the chiropractor showed me. I was amazed that I had never noticed any of it before. In my 16 years of searching for answers, no one had mentioned any of it to me. I was shocked to realize how far off my body was. Of course I was in pain! My whole spine was out of alignment.

I started to understand what a leg length discrepancy was and why it might be the cause of my pain. I started doing research and found there are two types of leg length issues.

Anatomical Short Leg

An anatomical short leg is when one leg is actually physically shorter than the other. The lengths of the bones are different. It is a skeletal problem that could have come from a birth defect or it could have resulted from a surgery. A hip or knee replacement could cause a short leg. I am told that it is very rare to have an anatomical short leg.

Non-Anatomical Short Leg

If you have a non-anatomical short leg, then one of your legs is not actually physically shorter than your other leg. Instead, the shortness of the leg comes from a rotation of the pelvis or the spine, which is caused by some sort of muscle or ligament issues. It is a non-skeletal problem and it is the most common type of short leg. Certain tests can be used to determine which type of short leg you have.

I learned that I have a non-anatomical short leg. It was interesting to me to learn that the short leg diagnosis has been around for a very, very long time; it is by no means a recent phenomenon. The typical treatment for a short leg is a heel lift, which is just a spacer of a certain thickness that is placed under the heel of the foot in the shoe. The standard thickness is 3/8".

George Evans showed me that what the heel lift tries to do is put your whole body back into alignment. To help me see how far out of alignment my body was, he showed me how to look at my pelvis.

There are two bony protrusions on the pelvis that make up the anterior superior iliac spine, or *ASIS*.

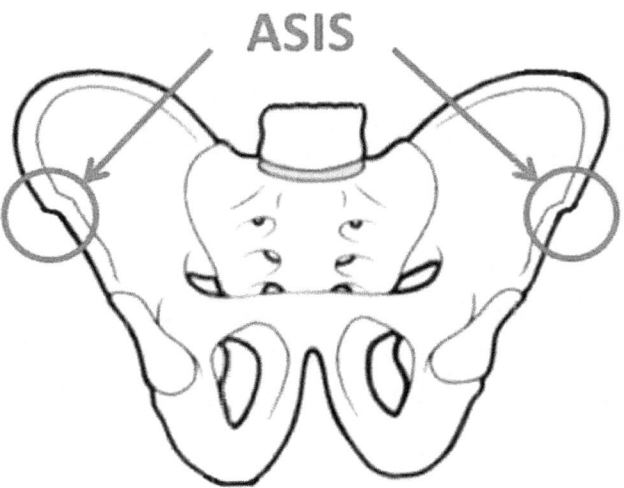

Figure 3

George taught me how to stand and place my fingers on my ASIS to determine how much rotation my pelvis has. It is a pretty simple process: I place my index fingers parallel to the ground and look down to see if one side is farther forward than the other. Turns out, a short right leg causes the right side of the pelvis to be lower and rotated forward, and vice versa. Makes perfect sense.

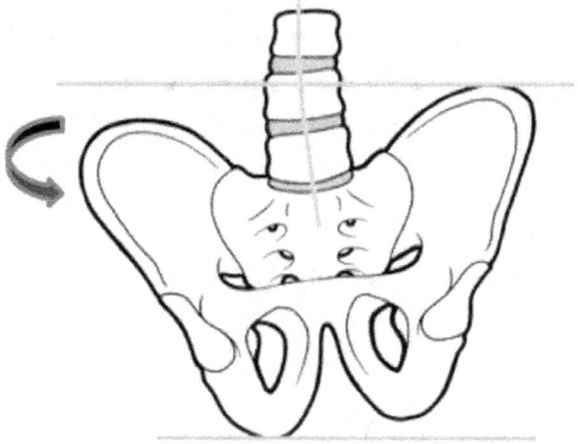

Figure 4

Once I determined how far off my pelvis was, it was easy to figure out how I could correct it. By placing a heel lift under my right foot, I could put my pelvis back into alignment. I could even place two heel lifts under my right foot and create a short left leg. I tried it and confirmed that my left pelvis was lower and rotated forward. By placing my hands on my ASIS, I could determine precisely how much correction my body needed.

With George's instruction, I began to understand for the first time exactly what my short leg was doing to my body. It was the cause of my body getting out of alignment. It also explained why my pelvis, shoulders, and head were not straight and level.

Armed with this helpful information, I committed myself to wearing a heel lift full time. But the solution was not foolproof: I'd only get the benefits of the correction while I was standing with my shoes on. As soon as I took my shoes off, there went the correction.

I added a heel lift to a pair of my slippers so that I'd get the correction when I was walking around the house Even if I got up to go to the bathroom in the middle of the night, I'd put on my slippers. Once I starting correcting my alignment, I'd know whenever my body was misaligned since the pain would intensify immediately. I could no longer go without the correction; I was forced to wear the heel lift whenever I was standing upright.

A problem arose when I sat down because the heel lift would only raise the lower part of my leg and that did me no good. When I was sitting, the pain would just get significantly worse again. That meant I was forced to stand as much as possible.

I needed some correction while I was sitting.

Since I knew how to measure my alignment while I was standing, I used the same method to determine my alignment while I was sitting down. I'd look at myself in a mirror and, if my shoulders were not level, it meant that my ASIS was out of alignment. The amount that it was off just happened to be equivalent to the amount that I'd be out of alignment while I was standing without a heel lift. In other words, I had the exact same problem sitting that I had standing. This explained why my pain increased when sitting. My pelvis was rotating out of alignment every time I sat down. I needed a way to place my pelvis into proper alignment when I sat down.

I discussed my idea with George and he told me about something called an *ischial tuberosity lift*. It's a pad of the same thickness as a heel lift that is placed under the ischial tuberosity (the sit bone) that puts the pelvis back into alignment. So I tried it for a while and I did find a small amount of relief. I'd just carry around a magazine and every time I sat down, I'd place it under my right sit bone.

Unfortunately, I discovered a big problem with the ischial tuberosity lift. The right side of my pelvis was not only lower but it was also rotated forward. The ischial tuberosity lift only addressed the height issue; it did not address the rotation. I needed to lift the right side and push my left gluteus maximus forward at the same time. That meant that when I sat down, I needed two magazines: one to go under my right sit bone and lift it and the other placed just so to push the left side of my pelvis forward.

I realized that magazines had their limits and they weren't going to work for me anymore. I had to design a product that would deliver both of the corrections I needed at any time I wanted to sit down.

I purchased a product that looked something like a tractor seat and was designed to support the pelvis. I modified it by adding a couple of pads. One pad went under the sit bone and the other pad pushed on the gluteus maximus.

Figure 5 - One pad lifts one side of the pelvis while the other rotates the pelvis back into alignment.

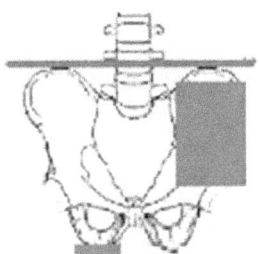

It worked. When I sat down and looked at myself in the mirror, I saw that my body was in perfect alignment.

Just as I did with standing, I found I needed constant correction while I was sitting. Sitting without correction would instantly cause my pain to skyrocket. My body was starting to calm down now that I was no longer out of alignment all the time. I was getting regular massages and my muscles were not as tight as they once were. My ability to sit down longer had greatly increased. Sitting in the car was now manageable. Things were starting to improve.

The problem with my homemade solution was that it was quite large. I had to carry it around in a backpack and pull it out every time that I wanted to sit down. It was not very convenient. I needed a better solution.

Larkin Lift

I decided I wanted to design a product that I could wear. That way, I'd always have correction available to me and I wouldn't need to carry anything around with me. Using a standard undergarment and pads that were made out of felt, I began to experiment. After some trial and error, I determined that the pads should be the same thickness as the heel lift. I sewed several pieces of felt together to get the right thickness and after figuring out where the pads should go, I sewed them in place.

I discovered that in order to engage the gluteus maximus pad and rotate my pelvis; I had to sit with my lower back against a chair back so it would push my pelvis into alignment. So from then on, I would only sit in chairs that would properly correct my alignment. I wouldn't sit on my couch or any chair that did not have proper lower back support any more. If I couldn't find a chair with proper back support, then I wouldn't sit down; it was the only way I could get any pain relief. And, believe me, any improvement in pain makes a big difference.

I was starting to feel better. I had designed a wearable posture-correcting device for myself. I called it the Larkin Lift and got it patented. I worked with a seamstress to design several pair and I wore them every day. I also found that the Larkin Lift placed my pelvis into a neutral position even when I lied down on my back. The gluteus maximus pad was rotating my pelvis while lying down. It was an added benefit that I didn't even plan on.

My product worked perfectly: every time I sat down, I had correction. The length of time I was able to sit down dramatically increased. And it was great to not have to carry something around. My life was beginning to change. People started noticing that I was feeling better. Someone told me I had a smile on my face for the first time in a long time. I had been in so much pain for so long that smiling had not been an option.

I had made some great strides, but my journey to great health wasn't over. Even with my posture correction devices, my back would still rotate and slip out of alignment frequently. Almost any movement would cause my spine to dislocate and then it would stay stuck that way. So I still needed to go to the chiropractor a lot. There was still a piece of the puzzle that I was missing.

Chapter 4
Chiropractic Care

I was desperate to figure out why I still needed constant chiropractic care even though my back was in proper alignment. I wanted to learn what chiropractors actually do when they treat people since they were providing the only treatment method that was helping me function at all. Here's what I learned:

Chiropractors treat what they call a *vertebral subluxation.* Wikipedia defines it this way:

> *In chiropractic, vertebral subluxation is a supposed misalignment of the spinal column leading to a set of signs and symptoms sometimes termed vertebral subluxation complex.*

Basically, a subluxation is a partial dislocation, misalignment, or over-rotation of one or more vertebrae in the spine. According to chiropractors, just a small amount of dislocation can cause neurological irritation, which causes pain. The figure below shows a chiropractic subluxation.

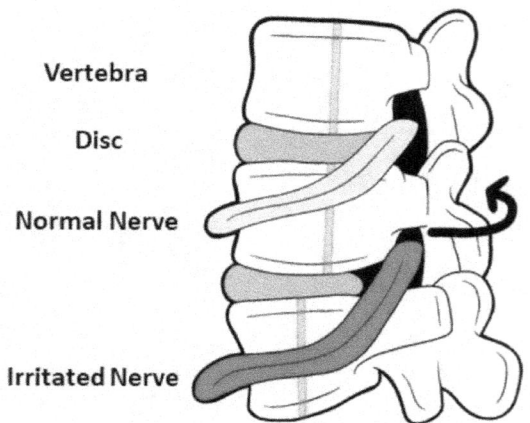

Figure 6 - Subluxation occurs when the spine is partially dislocated, causing irritation to the nerve

So how does a chiropractor determine if a person has a dislocated spine? They simply do a visual inspection. Just like the ASIS on the front of the pelvis, there are two protrusions on the back of the pelvis called the *PSIS*, short for posterior superior iliac spine. Chiropractors have their patients lie down on a table and then look at their PSIS to determine if there is a misalignment. They can also look at the facets of the spine to determine if there's a misalignment. They are very skilled at looking at these misalignments and can quickly determine if a vertebra or the pelvis is off.

Once a chiropractor determines the nature of the dislocation, they can treat the problem. They can apply a force to rotate the spine back into alignment. They might be able to press directly on a joint to make it move. If not, they might be able to use a person's legs to create more torque, which helps to move the joint. They have several different techniques to adjust the spine and most highly skilled chiropractors can put a joint back into alignment with only one or two tries. The act of placing the spine back into alignment is called *spinal manipulation*. The whole process doesn't take much time. A person can get in and out of a chiropractor's office in a matter of minutes.

I noticed that my spine was in either one of two states, depending upon whether I had subluxation or not. When I did, my back pain was pure torture. I'd literally count the seconds until I could see my chiropractor and get my spine put back into alignment. Until that happened, I'd put my life on hold. If I couldn't get to the chiropractor immediately, I'd lie down somewhere because any other activity, including sitting and standing, was just too painful.

Then I noticed that almost every time I dislocated my spine, I heard a pop. I became like Pavlov's dogs: any time I heard a pop, I'd cringe because I knew the pain was on its way.

I plotted a chart showing the level of pain I was experienced over a seven-year period, from when I first hurt my back, until I started to get regular chiropractic treatments. As you can see, I lived with a very high level of pain.

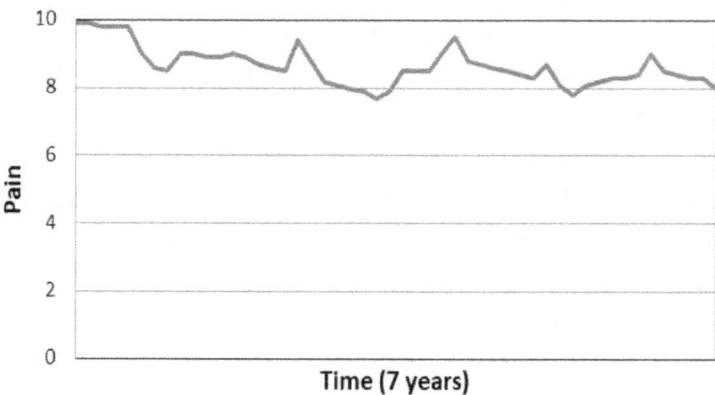

Figure 7

I continued plotting my pain levels for the next seven years when I was receiving regular chiropractic treatments. It might look like the chart makes absolutely no sense.

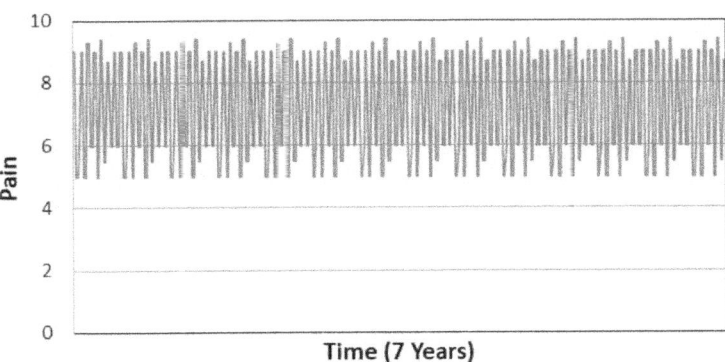

Figure 8

But if you zoom in, you see that my pain spiked every time I had a subluxation, and then it would drop back down after I got an adjustment with the chiropractor.

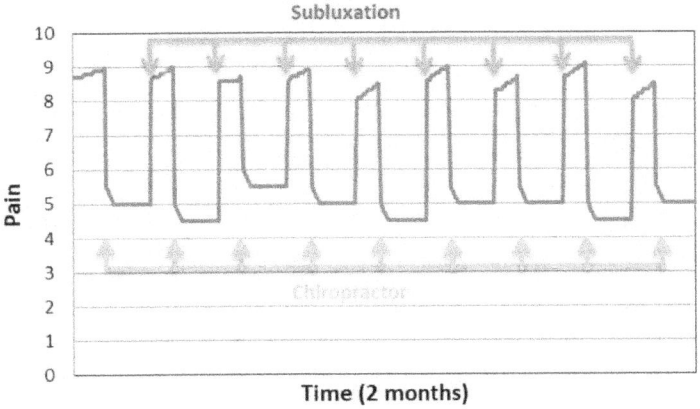

Figure 9

The chart in Figure 8 shows how many fluctuations I was going through: at least 60 chiropractic visits per year. I probably could have used an adjustment every day, but I was limited by my health insurance and out-of-pocket costs. If I had a subluxation on a Friday night, I'd spend the entire weekend in pain lying on the couch. I lost a lot of weekends of my life due to subluxations. I did not know what was causing them, but I did know that without chiropractic care, I'd probably be dead. It was the only thing that kept me functioning.

By the way, the degree of pain I was in also varied a lot based on what part of my spine the subluxation had occurred. Any subluxation was painful, but a subluxation in my lower back or pelvis was the most painful by far. My neck also required constant manipulation and was always in severe pain.

Subluxation Pain

So why is a subluxation so horrifically painful?

Let's look at the function of the spine. The vertebrae are stacked on top of each other and they're designed to pivot and rotate relative to each other. Each vertebra has a small range of motion relative to the adjacent vertebra. The cumulative effect of all the vertebrae creates a large range of motion. At the same time, all movement is limited by the facets, ligaments, and fascia.

A subluxation is an over-rotation of the vertebra; the joint has rotated past its normal range of motion and has become stuck in that position. In addition, the ligaments can't do their job and return the joint to its correct position; they remain in a lengthened state themselves. This is an abnormal state for the spine that ultimately causes neurological irritation.

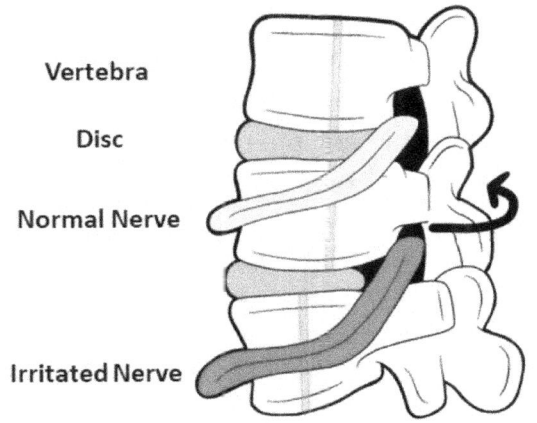

Figure 10 - In subluxation, a vertebra remains over-rotated and causes pain due to irritated nerves

It's important to recognize that a subluxation can initiate a viscious cycle of events that can very quickly escalate into a worsened condition, causing more and more pain. In engineering, the phrase *positive feedback loop* perfectly describes this effect. One condition feeds the next, which feeds the next, making the condition more entrenched as time goes on.

The positive feedback loop of subluxation begins with the vertebral misalignment, which causes the nerves to become irritated—which in turn causes the muscles to tighten. Once the muscles tighten, they continue to pull the verebrae out of alignment and the subluxation becomes more stuck. That, in turn, causes more neurological irritation, and so on. The pain increases and the condition continues to worsen very quickly.

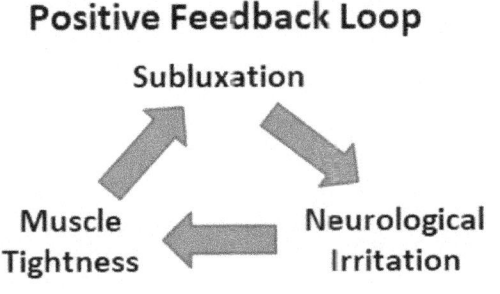

Figure 11- The viscious cycle of subluxation, neurological irritation and muscle tightness

Because of the cumulative effect of the positive feedback loop that my spine was stuck in, I was in a lot of pain. I sought help by getting chiropractic adjustments, where they apply enough force to rotate the spine back into its proper position. As a result, the positive feedback loop would get interrupted, and the pain would reduce. At least until the next subluxation occurred.

What makes matters worse is that when a dislocation occurs, it primarily affects nerves on only one side of the body. As a result, pain travels down one leg and causes muscles on that one side to become tighter. The muscle imbalance then feeds the positive feedback loop, making the condition more entrenched.

I lived many years of my life stuck in that painful loop of subluxation. Besides the neurological pain, my muscles got locked up tight, which is painful in and of itself. I spent a lot of money on massage just trying to get a little relief from that. But massage only provided some temporary relief because it only addressed the muscle tightness; it did not correct the subluxation and it did not stop the positive feedback loop. And since my body was constantly reacting to the pain by tightening up my muscles, it wouldn't take long after a massage before they'd be tight all over again.

As long as I treated the subluxation right away, I could survive when my muscles weren't quite so tight. The tightness decreased because I was able to shut down the positive feedback loop for small periods of time. My body was able to relax until the next subluxation occurred. I also required less massage and the massage I was getting worked more effectively.

The chart below shows all of the areas of my spine that could dislocate and require chiropractic manipulation. They wouldn't necessarily all be out every time I went to a chiropractor, but several areas would be dislocated, causing pain, and needing chiropractic adjustment.

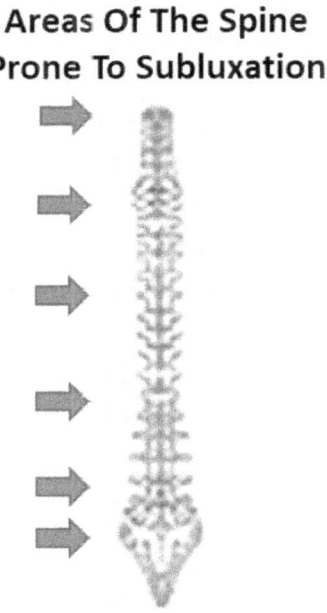

Figure 12

I was experiencing subluxations in my neck, upper back, lower back, and sacrum. Every time I went to the chiropractor, all four areas would have to be checked. With so many areas prone to subluxation, one area was always dislocated. And of course that meant I always had some muscles that were constantly being irritated. Even with frequent chiropractic visits, I was always in pain.

Types of Neurological Pain

You might think that neurological pain is only produced in those areas where a subluxation occurs, but it is not the case. I've found that there are two types of neurological irritations that occur, resulting in pain. The first type occurs at the point of the vertebral shift. This assymetrical shift causes pain to radiate outward through the path of the nerve on one side of the body only. The pain may be worse where the nerve directly exits the spine, but it may also travel down the entire length of the nerve. This would be the cause of sciatica. This type of pain has been well documented. There are spinal nerve charts that show the areas of the body that each nerve serves. There are also dermatome charts that show the areas of the skin that each nerve serves. These charts are very helpful to determine what area of the spine may be the cause of pain.

But there's another type of neurological irritation that is present when a subluxation occurs. It's when the nerves inside the spinal canal are also irritated, causing pain to radiate both upwards and downwards in the spinal canal. When I first hurt my back, I couldn't understand why I couldn't pinpoint the exact location of my pain. The best I could do was to point to an area of my spine and say that my pain was somewhere "around there." Now I understand that I couldn't pinpoint the exact location because pain was traveling both upwards and downwards in my spine, making it impossible to determine a precise location. Because I couldn't provide an exact location, it became an impossible problem to solve. My treatment method was left to imaging studies and opinions.

So how do I know this second type of neurological pain exists? I have been through hundreds and hundreds of subluxation correction cycles. Every time that I had a subluxation, I'd observe the pain that I was having. I could dislocate my lower back only and my neck would also be in pain. Pain was traveling up my spinal canal to my neck. Once I treated my lower back, my neck pain would go away.

The entire spine is affected when any area of the spine is dislocated. The pain is just more pronounced at the spot where the dislocation occurs. This second type of neurological pain is only present when the first type of neurological pain is present. I have also talked to chiropractors and found that chiropractors themselves cannot pinpoint what segment of their spine is causing pain when they have a subluxation. It just confirms that they also have this type of pain.

I find it interesting that our muscles aren't the only things affected when a subluxation occurs. Anything that is also controlled by the nerve is affected. For example, the intense pain I'd get from a dislocation would suppress my appetite. But after an adjustment, I'd immediately get my appetite back. The mechanism suppressing my appetite would go away when my dislocation was corrected.

Chapter 5
A Structural Analysis

Even though I was beginning to understand what chiropractors do to treat people, I wasn't any closer to solving my problem of chronic back pain. So I decided to learn more about what happens to my body when my spine has a subluxation. And, as an engineer, I couldn't help but look at it from a structural engineering perspective. This is how I began to see it:

If you take a structure that is not designed to rotate, and you rotate it, it will lose its structural integrity, and deformation will result. For example, imagine a soda can. Now, imagine it as two vertebrae with a disc in between.

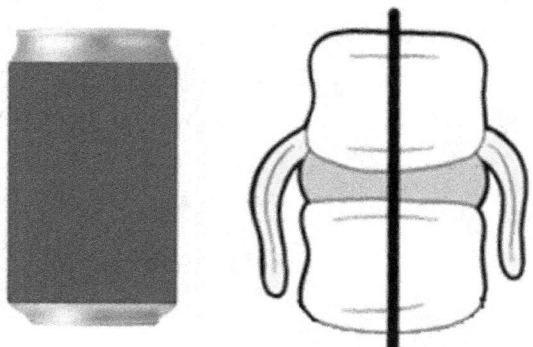

Figure 13

If you grab the top and the bottom of the can and twist them in a way that's similar to the action of a subluxation, two things will happen to it. First, it will wrinkle due to the rotation. Second,

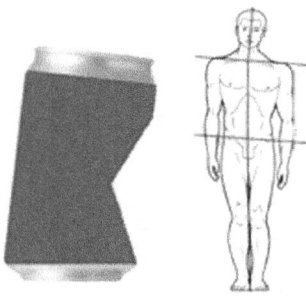

the top of the can will no longer be in vertical alignment with the bottom of the can.

Figure 14 - Try to rotate a structure that's not designed for rotation and misalignment results

In essence, the can has structurally failed. It can no longer support the same amount of load that it originally could. Due to the twist we gave the can, the top and the bottom of the can is no longer in alignment—which is exactly what happened to my spine.

I could see that my pelvis, shoulders, and head were no longer level. They were leaning to one side. I began to understand that, while my spine allows a small amount of rotation, as long as one of my vertebrae is rotated beyond its normal range of motion, then each and every vertebra above the area of dislocation becomes tilted along with it.

Figure 15 - Subluxation causes all of the vertebrae above the rotation to tilt to one side

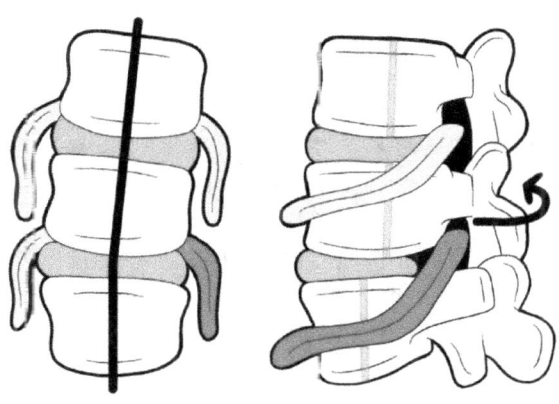

My spine was acting just like the soda can. The failure mechanism was identical. And the wrinkles that showed up in the can manifested as a disc bulge in my spine.

This explains why my back was so crooked. A subluxation by definition is a dislocation of the spine; that results in a structural failure.

Here is what is really interesting. There is a limit to how far the spine can rotate when it is dislocated. The structure of the spine only allows a small amount of movement. The range of movement for a single vertebra appears to be around 1/8" or so. As a result, it only takes a small shift to create neurological irritation.

My body would get affected differently depending upon where the dislocation of my spine occurred. If the lowest vertebra of my spine was dislocated, my pelvis would also rotate, creating a short leg. That meant that the small shift in my lower back would be translated through my pelvis, resulting in a rotation that was larger in effect than the original rotation. In other words, a 1/8" shift in my lower back now caused a 3/8" leg length discrepancy.

A dislocation higher up in my spine would have less of an effect on my pelvis. A dislocation in my upper back didn't rotate my pelvis but did rotate my shoulder forward. The same thing occurred in my neck. A dislocation high up in my neck would rotate my neck only and not my shoulders.

There was one more area of my spine that would also dislocate: my sacrum.

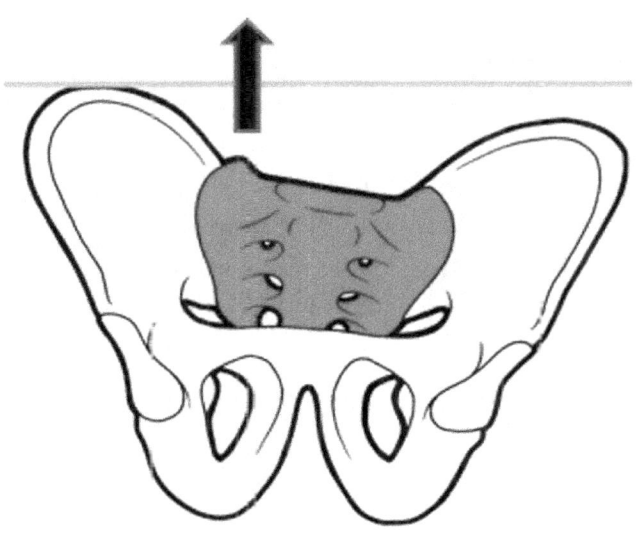

Figure 16 - A short leg eventually causes the sacrum to shift up on the opposite side.

My short leg condition would cause my pelvis to tilt to one side, and that in turn would exert a large amount of force on my sacrum. As a result, my sacrum eventually shifted upward on the other side of my pelvis. My chiropractor would treat the dislocation of my sacrum with a *drop table*, a table that has a section that literally drops, allowing for an adjustment without a twisting motion. He would press on my sacrum and the table would fall by a small amount, creating a large force that would help push my sacrum back into alignment.

While a vertebral subluxation usually caused a 3/8" leg length discrepancy, a sacrum dislocation caused an even bigger disparity in my leg length—by as much as 1" once my sacrum dislocated.

Armed with this new information, I had become a posture expert. I knew which area of my spine was dislocated by the amount of my leg length discrepancy. I could now walk into a chiropractor's office and tell them exactly what area of my spine was dislocated. I could also look at other people and determine if they had leg length issues. Once I started looking, it became very easy to spot other people with postural issues. I could also determine if they had dislocated their sacrum. These people are very easy to identify because their shoulders are nowhere near level, they lose the ability to sit down, and they require frequent position changes because of the constant pain.

Loaded vs. Unloaded Spine

Even though I had gained a lot of knowledge about my posture, I was still no closer to solving my back issue. I still needed to wear posture correction devices and I still needed endless amounts of chiropractic adjustments. But, I started to understand why my posture was partly to blame for my need for constant chiropractic care.

I also discovered something strange when I went to my chiropractor. When I walked in with a subluxation, and with my pelvis out of alignment to some degree, the chiropractor would adjust me and then tell me that my spine was back in alignment. But when I looked at myself in the mirror while standing up, I could see that my pelvis was still off—just by a smaller amount. The chiropractor believed that I was in alignment but it was clearly not so. Even after an adjustment, I still needed a heel lift to place my spine into proper alignment. In theory, I should have been in perfect alignment, but I wasn't. What was going on?

I realized that there was a fundamental difference between what I was doing to evaluate my posture and what my chiropractor was doing. Yes, we were looking at the same body, but we were looking at it literally from two different perspectives. I was looking at the alignment of my spine when I was in a standing position; my chiropractor was looking at it when I was lying down. And the two perspectives returned different results.

Another piece of the puzzle started to become clear. After a chiropractic adjustment, and while I was still lying on the table, my entire back was perfectly aligned. But if I looked at myself in the mirror while standing up, I easily recognized areas that were not lined up properly anymore. It seemed logical that it had something to do with the fact that the prone position put no weight on my spine from above. But, if I stood up, the weight of my upper body would bear down on my spine, and for some reason, my pelvis would then register a small rotation. But I didn't have an explanation for it. I had to keep digging.

Chapter 6
PRP

I had finally discovered that my pain was due to a structural failure of my spine—but I didn't know how to treat it. It was also obvious to me that, among all the doctors and practitioners I had seen in my journey to wellness, no one knew how to treat the structural failure, either. Everyone seemed willing to give me a diagnosis; but no one ever was able to give me a treatment that worked. It was up to me to solve the problem.

I had heard from a couple of people that the condition of my ligaments could be the cause of my chronic, debilitating pain. Now, I had tried prolotherapy to repair my ligaments before but the process had been absolutely useless to me. I had spent a lot of money on it, too, and I saw no improvement in my health.

I discovered a new treatment method called *Platelet Rich Plasma* (PRP), which is an adaptation of prolotherapy. Instead of injecting ligaments with an irritant solution, a person's own concentrated blood is used. Blood is taken from the patient and injected into seven or eight ligaments in order to promote healing of the ligaments.

I was desperate for real pain relief, so I decided to try the procedure. Of course, my insurance didn't pay for it so the cost was all out of pocket for me. It's only money, right? I also opted to have Human Growth Hormone (HGH) added to the injection, which increased the cost even more. My situation was so unstable and I felt so vulnerable to another onslaught of pain that I had nothing to lose.

First Injections

I was having a lot of pain near my coccyx so I decided to target that area for the injections first. I was hoping to get the injections in the ligaments to the left of my sacrum, but the doctor decided to do most of the injections further down, near my coccyx. She only did one or two injections into my ligaments. The whole procedure was fairly quick. Post-treatment, I was told to apply heat and avoid any bending or lifting. I drove home and sat on the couch for a week. I was so anxious for this procedure to work that I was super careful with bending and lifting.

Unfortunately, soon after I received the PRP treatment, I pulled another part of my spine out of alignment so I needed to get off the couch, get in my car, and go see a chiropractor again. As I drove to the chiropractor's office, I noticed that I was having trouble sitting. The pain was worse than usual. Even with my posture-correction devices in place, I couldn't sit down for very long. The injections had apparently caused a change to my body but it seemed like it made me worse, not better. I avoided driving my car for another week and my pain calmed down. At that point, it was hard to tell if there was any improvement from the procedure at all.

Second Injections

The PRP injections could only be done once a month, so I had plenty of time to decide if I wanted to do more. Since my pain was still pretty severe, I didn't feel like I had any choice but to go ahead and do more. I decided that the next time I did the procedure; I would get the injections in my lower back. Responding to my request, the doctor started at the lowest segment of my spine and worked her way up. She was able to inject four segments. I felt an intense pain for a couple of minutes, but then the pain calmed down. I went home and laid down for the rest of the day.

When I woke up the next morning, I looked at myself in the mirror. Something truly remarkable had happened. My pelvis, shoulders, and head were all in alignment. I no longer needed a heel lift while standing. In this Aha moment, I knew that the reason I was finally in alignment was because I had fixed my damaged ligaments.

A ligament is a band of dense connective tissue whose job it is to connect bones to bones. If a ligament is damaged, it can't be counted on to keep bones in their proper alignment and place.

I figured I knew something that no one else on the planet knew: the cause of chronic back pain is ligament damage. The medical term for ligament damage is *ligament laxity*. My conclusion explained why I needed so much chiropractic care: My damaged ligaments could no longer provide the structural support my spine needed to keep the joint from moving beyond its normal, healthy range. And almost any movement would allow my spine to move beyond the safe zone and get dislocated.

What amazed me was that I not only knew the cause of chronic back pain but I also knew the cure. PRP fixes ligament laxity. Once the ligaments are fixed, the joint becomes structurally sound again. I knew at that moment that I had the power to change medicine forever.

My attitude completely changed. I continued to look at myself in the mirror, day after day, and I was amazed that I was still standing straight. I just could not believe how level I was. I also knew that it would take some time for my pain to calm down completely.

Over the next month, I found that if I moved a wrong way or pulled on something too hard, I would get a jolt of pain. It seemed to me that my ligaments instantaneously shortened, as they should, but my body had not adapted to the ligament change. The sensation slowly went away and I continued to maintain my alignment. Just stabilizing my lower back caused my quality of life to improve. My quality of life was now all the way up to a 3.

I still needed chiropractic adjustments on other parts of my body, but I avoided any adjustment of my lower back. I absolutely didn't want to disrupt the PRP healing process. I would ask the chiropractor to look at the alignment of my lower back just to see if it was dislocated. But every time that I went to the chiropractor, my lower back was always in perfect alignment. It never needed an adjustment again. The chiropractor would adjust my sacrum, upper back, and neck only.

More Injections

While I finally had the mechanism to fix my back, I still had a other areas that needed to be fixed. It was going to take a lot of injections and it was going to cost a lot of money. But none of it mattered because I was sure that if I could fix one area of my spine, I could fix all of the other areas of my spine as well. My only goal was to rid myself of chronic pain.

Since my lower back was staying in alignment, I decided to get some more injections into my left sacrum again. The left-sided coccyx pain was not going away. Again, the doctor decided to do most of the injections near my coccyx and just a couple into the ligaments of my sacrum. My response this time was nowhere near the response that I had with my lower back injections. I had hoped for a slam-dunk of a response, but I didn't get it. I did seem to feel a little better and I was a little more stable. There was a very small improvement.

A couple of weeks later, I was working around my house and did something that required me to push with my legs. By the time I was done, I was in horrible pain all over again. My sacrum had shifted and I needed to see the chiropractor. I had seemed to go back into an unstable state again. It seemed as if I had undone any improvement that I had gained from the injections into my sacrum. I could not explain why it had occurred at this point. But there was some great news. My lower back was staying in alignment. I didn't need to have it adjusted when I went to the chiropractor.

Solving my back pain for good was going to take some more trial and error.

I decided that I would do some injections into my right sacrum. I knew that my sacrum was shifting but I didn't know what ligaments were damaged. Maybe the right-sided ligaments were the problem, and not the left. I had the doctor inject into the ligaments on the right side of my sacrum only. I didn't have the response that I had with my lower back. Once again, I didn't achieve the outcome that I hoped for. I was beginning to think that maybe I didn't have the solution to my chronic back pain after all.

The whole time that I was trying to solve my back and sacrum issues, my neck was in incredible pain. I would wake up with a pain score of 7 and it would be a 9 by the end of the day. If I looked up for few minutes, my pain instantly increased. The pain was so bad that I decided to stop the sacrum injections and try some neck injections.

Neck Injections

My chiropractor had recommended that I get the lower part of the neck injected, so I had the doctor do that. Again, there was no significant improvement. It was all starting to piss me off. I started to feel that I was just wasting money on the injections. Why did I not get the same response that I got with my lower back?

Because my neck was in so much pain, I had no choice but to wait a month and then try the injections again. I didn't want to have the chiropractor adjust my neck, but because I was in pain, I had no choice. She adjusted both my upper and lower neck. Then, since there was obviously something wrong with my upper neck, I decided to get the next set of injections in my upper neck only. And something absolutely amazing happened. I had the exact same pain response that I had with my lower back. The very sharp and intense pain lasted a couple of minutes and indicated to me that the injected ligaments were damaged and that they were responding to the treatment. After that, my neck pain started to decrease. It was obvious to me that my upper neck was the cause of all my pain.

I was feeling much better by the third week, but I needed to go to the chiropractor for an adjustment. I made the mistake of letting him adjust my upper neck. My neck immediately went back into pain. It was similar to what I had experienced with my sacrum.

I was learning that if my ligaments were not given proper time to heal before an adjustment, then the positive effects of the PRP were neutralized. So essentially I had to start the process all over again. I only had to survive a week in horrible pain before I could have another injection.

One week later, I returned for another PRP treatment and received injections in my neck in exactly the same way as I had done four weeks before. From it, I had the same improvement as before. The PRP was definitely helping. I was able to last for another three weeks before I inadvertently jolted my neck while I was riding in someone's car and the pain started up all over again. I couldn't seem to maintain alignment in my neck, as I was able to do with my lower back, but at least I was getting some temporary pain relief.

Yet More Injections

Since only one segment of my neck was causing all of my pain, I decided to get PRP injections into multiple body parts on each visit. I began combining upper back injections with neck injections. My plan was to beat my neck into submission along the way.

I decided to modify my strategy for getting the injections. I was motivated to change things up because the injections were expensive and I was tired of wasting both time and money by injecting in places that weren't getting any results. So, instead of letting my doctor decide where to inject, I told her exactly where I wanted them done.

First, I'd go to see my chiropractor, get his help figuring out what segments of my spine were dislocated, and then have him do the adjustments to get my back into alignment. Then I'd immediately get the PRP injections. It made sense to me that if my ligaments were damaged, then restoring my spine to its most neutral position before getting injections would facilitate the greatest amount of ligament recovery. It didn't make sense to try and repair ligaments that were already under strain. In fact, it seemed absolutely insane to me that anyone would do it any other way. But my PRP doctor didn't care what position my spine was in before she did the injections. She was only interested in doing them.

My strategy worked. After a few more injections into my upper back and neck, I decided to inject my left sacrum again. I purposely avoided telling the doctor where my pain was and I had her only inject the ligaments on the left of my sacrum. The result was that I had the same sharp intense pain response that I had with my lower back. I knew at that moment that these ligaments were the cause of my pain.

Holy crap, I did it. I fixed my sacrum.

After a couple weeks of recovery, I went to the gym. I noticed that I could squat down all the way for the first time in a long, long time. Before the injections, something seemed to bind up and prevent me from squatting down. But now, my body was beginning to change. Things were improving. When I got a massage, it was even pleasant because my muscles were relaxed. After a couple of months, I felt a big improvement.

I had to replace the main water line to my house, which would require me to do things that I had not done in a very long time. Things like shoveling, bending, and lifting large stones had not been a part of my lifestyle for years. But I was able to do them and I was amazed at how good I felt. My sacrum didn't go out of alignment. My chiropractor even verified that I was in perfect alignment and no adjustment was needed.

I had done it. I had stabilized my neck, lower back and my sacrum. I had reached a major milestone. The best part was that I learned to do it on my own. My quality of life had lifted all the way to a 6.

There was only one more area of my back that was still having problems: my upper back. I could pull on something and it would dislocate. I was certain that I could fix that problem also. All that was needed was a little more trial and error.

By this time, when I went to see my chiropractor, he only adjusted my upper back. I would not even let him touch any other part of my spine. I knew it was in alignment and I didn't want to take the chance that he would screw up everything that I had done with PRP.

Since I only had one area of my spine that needed adjustment anymore, I tried to figure out how I could adjust it on my own. I designed a device that I could lie on to adjust my back without the help of a chiropractor. The good news was that I was able to do it my own. The bad news was that I was adjusting it two or three times a day. But because I had learned how to adjust it on my own, I stopped going to the chiropractor. I canceled my monthly plan. To cancel chiropractic care was another major milestone in my health progression. I could now manage my spine care on my own.

After a couple of injections in my upper back, I still could not stabilize that area and keep it from dislocating. I knew that failure mechanism of my upper back was identical to the failure mechanism of my lower back, but my upper back was not improving. There had to be something else that I was missing.

So this is what I discovered.

When it came to my lower spine, I was able to use a posture-correcting device to place the lower vertebrae of my spine into a neutral position. With the help of chiropractic, I removed the subluxation and thus removed all the strain on my ligaments, which could then heal properly with PRP injections. Once they got healthy, they no longer allowed my back to come out of alignment again. But when it came to my upper spine, I wasn't able to use a posture correction device at all. My right shoulder was rotated forward, which pulled my spine even further out of alignment and created constant strain on my ligaments. The injections were not effective because of the constant strain.

I started wearing a posture-correcting device to pull my shoulders backward. I also did a lot of hot yoga. These two activities allowed my shoulder and upper back muscles to finally loosen and calm down. I decided to have one more injection into my upper back. My chiropractor helped me to identify which segments were giving me the most pain and the doctor then injected there. Once again, I immediately knew that the injections had worked because of my pain response. I had done it again. I fixed my upper back.

My quality of life was now a pleasant 7.

Chapter 7
Ligament Laxity

I understood that the reason I continued to have chronic pain was that my back had developed ligament laxity. My spine had failed structurally. I also understood how to fix the ligament laxity with PRP treatments.

But why hadn't a professional given me the diagnosis of ligament laxity? To answer that, we need to take a closer look at ligament laxity.

As I've mentioned, the ligaments provide all of the structural support for the joints in the body. They are designed to keep the motion of a joint within its healthy, proper range of motion.

According to Wikipedia:

Ligaments are viscoelastic. They gradually strain when under tension, and return to their original shape when the tension is removed. However, they cannot retain their original shape when extended past a certain point or for a prolonged period of time. This is one reason why dislocated joints must be set as quickly as possible: if the ligaments lengthen too much, then the joint will be weakened, becoming prone to future dislocations. Athletes, gymnasts, dancers, and martial artists perform stretching exercises to lengthen their ligaments, making their joints more supple.

So, when a subluxation occurs, the vertebral shift causes the ligaments to be stretched.

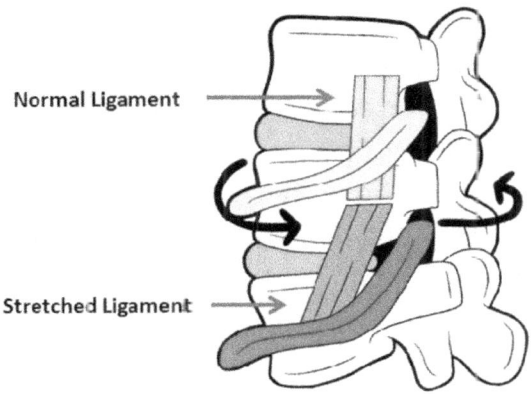

Figure 17 - A subluxation causes the ligaments to stretch

If the subluxation is not treated right away, the ligaments become lengthened and permanently damaged, and the joint is no longer structurally sound. Once the ligaments become lax, the joint gains freedom to move in—and out—of its proper, healthy position. The improper positioning is similar to the condition of a chain when there's extra movement, or play, where the links join together. It's what engineers call *backlash*, a weakness in the chain that makes it more susceptible to failure.

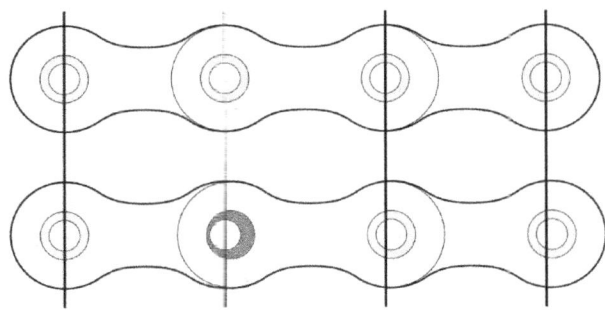

Figure 18 - Backlash in a chain link

From a mechanical viewpoint, backlash in a chain is a very bad situation. When a load is applied to the normal chain, the forces are distributed evenly. When a load is applied to a chain with backlash, the forces are no longer distributed equally. The load causes the chain to be pulled apart and makes it more susceptible to failure. The chain becomes structurally deficient. With the right amount of force, or more, the chain will pull apart and fail.

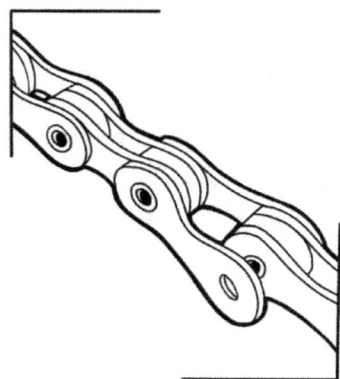

Figure 19 - When a chain has backlash, it can more easily pull apart and fail

The spine works in a similar fashion to the chain. Ligament laxity is the backlash and a subluxation is the failure. Once the ligaments have become damaged, the joint is not prevented from moving beyond its normal range, and the likelihood of a subluxation is greatly increased. That means a simple rotation of the spine can dislocate the joint. While a chain actually pulls apart and becomes unusable, the spine rotates into a position it can't back out of. And the dislocation then causes a lot of pain.

Extra Amount

Understanding ligament laxity helped me explain why there was a discrepancy between perceived misalignment in my back when I was standing versus when I was lying down. By standing up, my spine became loaded with the weight of my upper body, causing ligament laxity to become pronounced. When I laid down, the ligament laxity was no longer in play. Chiropractors never looked at me standing up. If they had, they would have seen that there was still a shift in my pelvis. My damaged ligaments were allowing my pelvis to shift slightly. Even when my back was in alignment, ligament laxity still created a rotated pelvis and a short leg.

From a neurological irritation point of view, ligament laxity is painful and a subluxation is very painful. Because of the ligament laxity in my back, every movement I made caused a neurological response. I was shifting into and out of positions that would apply a strain on my nerves. If the movement involved enough force, it would cause a subluxation to occur, get stuck there, and require a chiropractor to fix it. It explains why my health was so poor; my nervous system was constantly being irritated and my muscles locked up in response.

I often heard a popping sound when my spine went into subluxation or when my chiropractor adjusted my back. The prevailing theory is that small pockets of air that are suspended in fluid and that are popped during the adjustment create the popping noise. But I think that the ligaments are the cause of the sound. There has to be a reason why the spine gets into a stuck state. The ligaments are tough, rigid structures that are not designed to move. A subluxation forces the joint out of alignment. It would make sense that these ligaments move over other structures, such as other ligaments or bones, trapping the vertebrae in a stuck state—which is what the chiropractors are treating. The act of forcing the vertebra back into alignment causes the ligaments to snap back in place, thus creating a sound.

Once the ligaments are lax, the likelihood of a subluxation is greatly increased. Long, lax ligaments can easily move over other structures, causing the bones to become stuck. This explains why some people need frequent, ongoing chiropractic adjustments. Their spines are unstable due to ligament damage. While this is just my theory, it is amazing to me that once I fixed my ligament laxity issues, my spine no longer made popping noises or needed an adjustment.

Why Was This Not Diagnosed?

Over and over again, I'd ask myself why my ligament laxity had not been diagnosed. I finally had the answer. The gold standard for determining spinal issues is the MRI; In fact, an orthopedic surgeon will not see you without an MRI. But from the point of view of collecting data, there is an inherent flaw in the MRI procedure: they only do it with the patient lying down. As I've described, since the spine is in an unloaded position, any ligament laxity-related issues won't register. Even if the patient has a small shift of their vertebra from a subluxation, it will now become less pronounced because their spine is unloaded. Only small bulges in the discs will become visible. This shortcoming makes the MRI absolutely useless at detecting the pelvic or vertebral shift that indicates there's ligament laxity. The only way for an orthopedic surgeon to detect if ligament laxity is in play would be to do two MRIs: one while standing and one while lying down. The shift in the vertebrae, caused by ligament laxity, would then be able to be detected. No one in medicine even understands this.

Here's a surefire method that anyone can use to determine if they have ligament laxity. First, go to a chiropractor and have them rule out an anatomical short leg. Have them adjust you to get your spine in perfect alignment. Then stand up. If your pelvis is rotated, then the only explanation is that you have ligament laxity. Now look at your shoulders. If they are out of alignment, then there are two possible reasons. One is scoliosis. But if your chiropractor rules out scoliosis, then the only explanation is that you have ligament laxity. Just keep in mind that if you have scoliosis and you have chronic back pain, you could potentially have both scoliosis and ligament laxity.

Chapter 8
Muscle Imbalance

Once I had corrected my ligament laxity condition, you might think I would be back to normal and pain-free. Yet while removing the cause of the neurological irritation did reduce my pain a lot, I was by no means pain-free. I had one last problem to solve.

As I already described, a subluxation is an assymetrical rotation of the spine. This causes irritation to the nervous system on one side of the body only. These irritated nerves cause the muscles to become tighter and tighter on one side of the body only. This quickly creates a muscle imbalance, which in turn rotates the spine even further out of alignment. While one muscle is tightening up, the corresponding muscle lengthens to accommodate the first muscle. The longer a person is left in that state, the worse the muscle imbalance becomes.

Asymmetrical Muscle Imbalance Resulting From A Subluxation

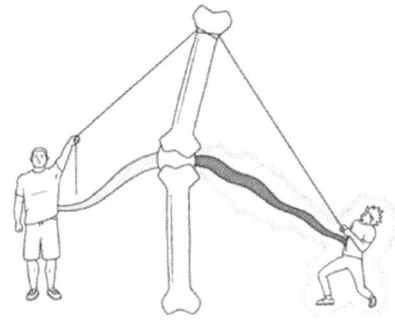

Figure 20

Over time, the muscles become stuck in their states. One muscle becomes stuck short and the other muscle becomes stuck long. Even if all of the causes of neurological irritation are removed, the muscles stay stuck and the spine remains predisposed to rotate out of alignment.

So what happens when a muscle gets tighter and tighter? After a while, a tight muscle passes a threshold from no pain to pain. Just taking a muscle and increasing its tightness sufficiently will produce pain. If you ever experienced a muscle cramp, you understand what an extremely tight muscle feels like.

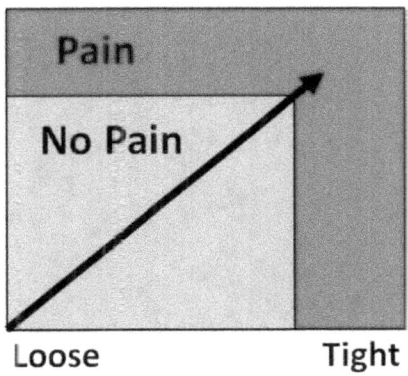

Figure 21

A subluxation works on a much lower threshold of pain than a cramp but the continuous neurological irritation causes the muscle to eventually become locked up and that becomes very painful. Just look at anyone with chronic back pain and you will find that their body is all seized up due to muscle tightness.

The real problem is that the longer a muscle is left in this tightened state, the weaker it becomes. It fatigues quickly and that causes more pain. While a healthy person can do a certain amount of work before their muscles tighten up, someone with chronic pain will reach their pain threshold much more quickly. Most people with chronic back pain never return to a normal healthy state because their muscles are weak and they fatigue easily.

One might also think that having a short leg would cause the muscles on only one side the body to tighten, but it's not the case.

Lines Of Force Due To Uneven Loading Of The Spine

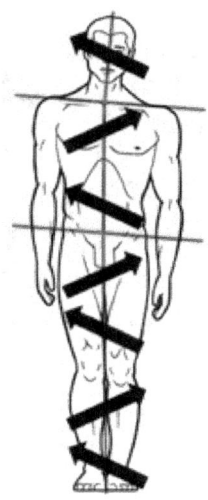

Figure 22

Once a short leg condition occurs, the entire body is affected, causing pain and muscle tightness to occur at different points on both sides of the body. First, the pelvis lowers on one side and also rotates forward on the side with the short leg. Then, like a chain reaction, the muscles adapt to the short leg and they do so asymmetrically; one rotation causes other rotations. I had pain in my right foot, left calf, left hamstring, right hip and back, left chest, right shoulder, and my neck was completely screwed.

Stuck States

The question then becomes what to do with the muscles that are in stuck states? Let's look at the individual muscles. Fixing the muscle that's stuck in the lengthened position is fairly easy. Simply strengthening it should return it to its normal state. There's nothing wrong with the muscle; it just hasn't been used because of the structural imbalance in the body. Once it gets used to working again, it quickly remembers its function, and it gets healthy again.

The shortened muscle, on the other hand, has a completely different problem. The shortened muscle needs strengthening, but it also has to be lengthened. You can strengthen a muscle by exercising it and you can lengthen a muscle by stretching it. Lengthening, however, is not an easy task because the muscle has become stuck where it is and fascia have grown around it, helping to keep it trapped in its condition. Also, the longer the muscle has been in that state, the harder it is to get it unstuck. It has to be coaxed to come out of its shortened state; it will not do it on its own.

Lengthening is a much harder and much slower process than strengthening. We'll discuss both in the next chapter.

Chapter 9
The Larkin Method

Once I developed a deep understanding of the cause of chronic back pain and its successful treatment, I put together a treatment plan to treat chronic back pain and reduce or eliminate the pain one suffers with. It is a multistep process that can be applied to any or all areas of the spine. These are the steps I followed to treat several areas of my spine and to return me to a pain-free life.

There are five steps to the process I created. Together, I call them *The Larkin Method*.

The Larkin Method

1	2	3	4	5
Correct Subluxations	Modify Posture	Loosen and Lengthen Muscles	Repair Ligaments	Correct Muscle Imbalance

Figure 23

If you are living with chronic back pain, I will show you how to correct your problem with The Larkin Method. The key to being successful will be to understand the cause of your pain. The more you learn about your body, the easier it will be to fix your problem and get yourself pain-free.

Keep in mind that solving your chronic back pain is not a simple process; it cannot be solved with a pill or one simple procedure. Do not expect instantaneous results. It involves work—

a lot of work. If you've been living with chronic back pain for years, it will take time to return to normal health.

There are several steps to my process. I highly recommend that you follow them in order.

Step 1 – Correct Subluxations

The goal of this step is to identify and correct the areas of your spine that are dislocated.

Chiropractors are highly skilled at identifying what areas of the spine are dislocated and treating them, so any time you go to a chiropractor, always ask which areas of your spine are dislocated. The information you get will be crucial to the next steps of the process. Begin to notice and measure what your pain is like before and after an adjustment. Once you gauge that, if at any time you dislocate your spine, get it corrected it immediately. Because you haven't treated any of the causes of the problem yet, it is likely that you'll need repeated chiropractic adjustments. Don't be afraid to see the chiropractor as much as possible.

Keeping your spine in alignment will allow your nervous system to be less susceptible to irritation. The muscles will begin to calm down and you'll be in less pain. Learn to identify which movements cause a subluxation in your back and avoid those activities throughout this process. The more you learn about your dysfunction throughout the process, the more it will benefit you.

Step 2 – Modify Posture

The goal of this step is to get your spine into proper alignment and remove the strain on your ligaments.

A "short leg" causes the entire spine to be out of alignment. The pelvis, shoulders, and neck will no longer be straight and level if you have a short leg. Your chiropractor can easily identify which leg is short. If you have a short leg, use a heel lift. Look in the mirror, and figure out exactly what you look like with and without a heel lift. You may need to adjust the size of the heel lift to align your spine correctly. If your sacrum has shifted, you'll need to use a wearable posture correction device when you're sitting down. If there's pain in your shoulders, you'll need to wear a device that will pull your shoulders back. The location of where the subluxation is occurring will dictate the type of correction you should be using. You should wear your correction devices as much as you possibly can.

It's time to become extremely aware of your posture. The posture correction devices are just temporary measures to help your body to get back into proper alignment. You'll only need to wear them for a short time to allow your nervous system to calm down, to help your muscles begin to relax, and to remove the strain off of your ligaments.

Again, because you haven't treated anything yet, it is very likely that you'll need repeated chiropractic adjustments. Go to your chiropractor as much as possible. The use of posture-correcting devices might reduce your need for chiropractic care, but if a subluxation occurs, be sure to treat it immediately.

As you begin this process, you'll start to notice a difference with and without posture correction and you'll begin to get a feel for how your poor posture is creating pain. You'll start to learn how to avoid any activity that increases your pain. It will be very helpful to you to be able to identify these triggers.

Step 3 – Loosen and Lengthen Muscles

The goal of this step is to remove the strain on your spine caused by tight muscles that have been stuck in shortened conditions. By correcting your posture, you have reduced the neurological irritation from the subluxation and corrected the strain on your ligaments. But you haven't done anything for your muscles yet. In order to get the best results, your muscles have to be coaxed to return to their normal, relaxed state. This will require work on your part, and involve pain.

Talk with a variety of people to find techniques that will loosen and lengthen your muscles. Don't be concerned with strengthening any muscles at this point; you only want to get your body out of its locked up state. Take some time with this step; try to eliminate as much muscle tension as possible. Just reducing your muscle tightness will help to reduce your pain. Here are the methods I recommend you try first:

Physical Therapy

Use physical therapy in any way that you can. This is the one part of your healthcare treatment that is covered by insurance, so soak up whatever benefit you can. Get a physical therapist to identify which muscles are the tightest ones. They are experts at identifying tight muscles and addressing the soft tissue issues. They can show you how to stretch your muscles effectively, too.

Some physical therapists can also perform dry needling, a technique that inserts a small needle into the trigger point of a muscle while an electrical stimulator pulses the muscle, causing it to relax. Use this or any technique that you can find to relax your tight muscles.

Your insurance coverage will run out much faster than your muscles will relax, so gather as much information as you can. You can take this information with you to other specialists that you'll see.

Massage

Massage is great for loosening very tight muscles. By itself, massage will not lengthen a muscle, but it will loosen it, allowing you stretch it. Stretching after a massage makes it even better. Always find out from your massage therapist which of your muscles are the tightest.

Most massage therapists like to work on the body symmetrically. Because you've got a muscle imbalance, this is no longer the best approach. Your goal is to remove the muscle imbalance, so just have them work on the parts of the body that are the tightest. That will release the strain from your muscles and help get your spine back into proper alignment. Attack your imbalance with a lot of massage. The downside with massage is that it is usually not covered by insurance. Be prepared to spend a lot of money.

Also, if you are having trouble getting a chiropractic adjustment, a massage before an adjustment will loosen the muscles allowing the spine to be manipulated more easily.

Hot Yoga

Of all the therapies that I could do on my own to relax my muscles, I found hot yoga to be the best. Trying to stretch a muscle at room temperature is almost impossible, but when a muscle is heated, it becomes much more pliable. With hot yoga, you'll easily notice a change in your flexibility.

There are a couple of downsides to hot yoga. The first is that it is an extremely slow process, so you should be prepared to do a lot of hot yoga. The second is that hot yoga is a full body approach and can only target some of your muscles. You'll need to spend extra time on your own stretching the tight muscles that hot yoga doesn't target.

I noticed one thing with hot yoga that I didn't notice with any other form of therapy. Hot yoga really changes people's lives. I have never heard as many success stories with any other treatment as I have with hot yoga. Stretching in a hot room creates a transformative process for the body.

Fascial Stretch Therapy

If you are having trouble stretching on your own, there are people who will help you stretch. Fascial stretch therapy is a hands-on approach to lengthening muscles. A therapist will move a joint or muscle in ways that you can't do on your own. Having someone stretch you is far superior to trying to stretch yourself. The downside is that it is not covered by insurance and it is expensive. But, if it increases your range of motion and jump-starts your stretching, then it is well worth it.

Again, it's worth repeating that because you haven't treated any underlying issues yet, you may still need ongoing chiropractic adjustments. Go see your chiropractor as much as possible.

There is no simple way to lengthen a muscle. If these techniques do not work for you, then try to find anything else on your own that will help. The more muscle imbalance you can remove, the greater the results you'll receive in the next step.

Step 4 – Repair Ligaments

The goal of this step is to repair your damaged ligaments.

Everything you've done up to this point was done to allow your body to return to its proper, aligned state with no muscle or ligament tension. You had to remove the strain on your ligaments so they could heal properly when it's time to get them treated. And now's that time.

To treat the ligaments, get Platelet Rich Plasma (PRP) injections. The injections will enable the ligaments to shorten and return to their normal state. The process brings structural stability back to your joints.

So how do you know where to do the injections? Since you've gotten information from your chiropractor about which areas of your spine have subluxations, you can tell your PRP doctor to inject the ligaments at those locations. If your spine is damaged in several areas, it will take several visits to treat them all. It might also take multiple injections at the same sites.

I recommend that you go to the chiropractor just before you go to get PRP injections to align the spine and remove as much tension as possible. The last thing you want to do is try to shorten your ligaments while your spine is out of alignment.

After you get the injections, stop all activity. No bending, no lifting, and no stretching. Take as much time off as you can. Avoid all strenuous activity. Do not see anyone who will touch your spine. Give your body time to heal.

Your body will need time to adapt to the changes to your ligaments provided by your PRP treatments. Go back to your previous activities slowly over time. Because your ligament laxity has been fixed, your nervous system will no longer be constantly irritated. You should feel a gradual improvement almost every day.

After PRP, stop seeing your chiropractor. Your ligaments have returned to their normal state and your joints are now strong. There should be no reason to have to ever have a spinal manipulation again. Do not let a chiropractor talk you into thinking you need regular adjustments. You do not need regular adjustments because your ligaments have been repaired.

You are not done yet. There is one last step.

Step 5 – Correct Muscle Imbalance

The goal of this step is to return your muscles to a strong but relaxed state.

At this point, you haven't yet addressed the condition of your weak muscles. That's because it doesn't make sense to try and strengthen a muscle that is constantly being irritated and weakened. While you've successfully removed the neurological irritation on your spine and now that your joints are strong, you still have to resolve your muscle imbalance, since it is still trying to rotate your spine. Plus, your weak muscles will fatigue easily and cause pain.

Because your tight muscles have been stuck in a shortened condition, correcting your muscle imbalance requires both strengthening and lengthening. Since we've already discussed lengthening your muscles in Step 3, let's go right into what it takes to strengthen them.

First, it's important that you understand the importance of strengthening your muscles. They are much weaker than the muscles of someone who has not lived with chronic pain. If you don't strengthen your weak muscles, you'll never be completely free of pain. Your muscles will easily fatigue and cause you pain. You cannot ignore this step. You have no choice.

Strengthening is actually a much faster process then lengthening, but it will require hard work on your part. It will also require that you endure a fair amount of pain. But it's worth it. Push yourself. If you are not sore, you are not working hard enough.

So how do you know which muscles to strengthen and what exercises to do? Go to a physical therapist and ask a lot of questions; that is their specialty. They can quickly identify your weak muscles and show you the best exercises to strengthen them. Start working with their exercises and then progress to more and more weight.

Be sure to target individual muscles for strengthening. Each and every muscle that has been affected by the subluxation has to be isolated and strengthened. Use a variety of exercises and get as much information from your physical therapist as you can. If you think you can just walk around the block and get better, you'll never get rid of your back pain. If you think you can just go to a gym and sit on an exercise bike, you'll never fully recover because you won't be targeting the individual muscles that are very weak.

If you don't want to work for it, you'll never see pain-free days. You have to work harder than your friends because they haven't been living in pain the way you have been. There is no other solution.

But there's more. Don't forget to lengthen your short muscles as you strengthen them. Do both: go to the gym and do hot yoga. Strengthen, lengthen, and repeat. You'll reach a point at which your health skyrockets. The stronger your muscles become, the more activities you'll be able to do without pain. You'll soon return to your normal life.

Your Insurance Isn't Enough

There's one more thing you need to understand if you're going to try and treat your own chronic back pain. Your health insurance will not even come close to covering the costs. As I've mentioned, some of the treatments are not covered by insurance. Those that are covered are limited in the number of treatments you can receive. The time you'll need to completely solve your back problem will exceed any coverage from your insurance. You just have to throw money at the problem. It will be worth it once your back pain goes away forever.

Chapter 10
The Real Solution

The question I kept asking myself was: *Why*? Why did I have to create my own method to treat my chronic back pain? After all, there's a huge network of doctors, surgeons, physical therapists, chiropractors, pain medicine specialists, neurologists and so on in this country, yet I still had to find the solution to my chronic back problem all on my own.

An even better question is, *Why was no one in healthcare even coming close to solving my chronic back pain?* We live in modern times and some of today's advances in medicine are nothing short of phenomenal. Yet, I lost 16 years of my life to chronic pain. Why could no one in the medical field help me?

In order to explain why I had to solve this issue on my own, we have to discuss the way different healthcare providers view subluxations. To do so, I have split the variety of healthcare providers we seek help from into two categories. The first group is primary medicine, which includes all of the practitioners who would be covered by your health insurance plan. This group includes doctors, surgeons, physical therapists, pain medicine specialists, and anyone else who you may visit in a hospital or emergency care center. They are the people you are most likely to see when you've got an injury. The second category is alternative medicine. These are the chiropractors, massage therapists, fascial stretch therapists, acupuncturists, and anyone else who's not in the primary medicine group who you'll go to for help. You won't find anyone in this category in a hospital and they may or may not be covered by your insurance.

Now let's talk about how these two worlds define subluxation. Let's start with a chiropractor's definition. Here is Wikipedia's description of it. You can also easily find it in medical textbooks. It's interesting, so try to read the whole thing:

> *In chiropractic, vertebral subluxation is a supposed misalignment of the spinal column leading to a set of signs and symptoms sometimes termed vertebral subluxation complex. It has no biomedical basis and is categorized as pseudoscientific by leading authorities. Traditionally, the "specific focus of chiropractic practice" is the chiropractic subluxation and historical chiropractic practice assumes that a vertebral subluxation or spinal joint dysfunction interferes with the body's function and its innate intelligence, as promulgated by D. D. Palmer, the inventor of chiropractic.*
>
> *Within the chiropractic tradition, a vertebral subluxation complex is believed to be a dysfunctional biomechanical spinal segment which actively alters neurological function, which in turn, is believed to lead to neuromusculoskeletal and visceral disorders. The WHO acknowledges this difference between the medical and chiropractic definitions of a subluxation: medical doctors only refer to "significant structural displacements" as subluxations, whereas chiropractors suggest that a dysfunctional segment, whether displaced significantly or not, should be referred to as a subluxation. This difference has been noted in the proceedings of the chiropractic profession's Mercy Center Consensus Conference: "The chiropractic profession refers to this concept as a 'subluxation'. This use of the word subluxation should not be confused with the term's precise anatomic usage, which considers only the anatomical relationships."*

The chiropractic vertebral subluxation complex has been a source of controversy since its inception in 1895 due to the lack of empirical evidence for its existence, its metaphysical origins, and claims of its far reaching effects on health and disease. Although some chiropractic associations and colleges support the concept of subluxation, many in the chiropractic profession reject it and shun the use of this term as a diagnosis. In the United States and in Canada the term nonallopathic lesion may be used in place of subluxation.

A 2009 review concluded that epidemiologic evidence does not support the chiropractic subluxation, concluding:

"No supportive evidence is found for the chiropractic subluxation being associated with any disease process or of creating suboptimal health conditions requiring intervention. Regardless of popular appeal, this leaves the subluxation construct in the realm of unsupported speculation. This lack of supportive evidence suggests the subluxation construct has no valid clinical applicability."

In 2015, 8 internationally accredited chiropractic colleges: AECC, WIOC, IFEC-Paris, IFEC-Toulouse, USD-Odense, UZ-Zurich, UJ-Johannesburg and Durban University of Technology made an open statement which included: "The teaching of the vertebral subluxation complex as a vitalistic construct that claims that it is the cause of disease is unsupported by evidence. Its inclusion in a modern chiropractic curriculum in anything other than an historic context is therefore inappropriate and unnecessary".

So, from a chiropractic viewpoint, a subluxation is a misalignment or partial dislocation of the spine. This misalignment alters neurological function and creates pain. Because there is no major structural damage to the joint, it can be manipulated back into alignment by a chiropractor. So far, so good.

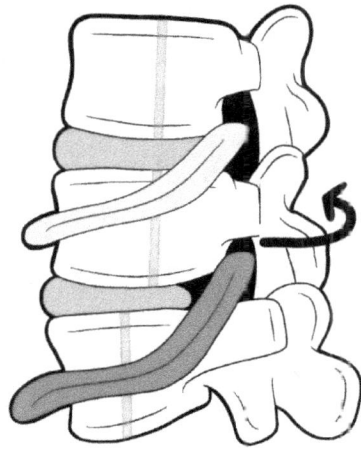

Figure 24 - A chiropractic subluxation is a misalignment of a vertebra

Now let's look at the definition of a subluxation as understood by medical doctors. In this case, it's called a *medical subluxation,* and here's Wikipedia's definition of it:

> *A subluxation may have different meanings, depending on the medical specialty involved. It implies the presence of an incomplete or partial dislocation of a joint or organ.*
>
> *An orthopedic subluxation of any joint will sometimes require medical attention to help relocate or reduce the joint. Nursemaid's elbow is the subluxation of the head of the radius from the annular ligament. Other joints that are prone to subluxations are the shoulders, fingers, kneecaps, ribs, wrists, ankles, and hips affected by hip dysplasia. A spinal subluxation can sometimes impinge on spinal nerve roots, causing symptoms in the areas served by those roots. In the spine, such a displacement may be caused by a fracture, spondylolisthesis, rheumatoid arthritis, severe osteoarthritis, falls, accidents and other traumas. This is common in Ehlers-Danlos Syndrome.*

At first, the medical definition of a subluxation appears to be the same as the chiropractic definition. But if you dig deeper, you see that the medical definition states that a medical subluxation only refers to a structural displacement *that is significant enough* to appear on static imaging studies. This is what a medical subluxation looks like.

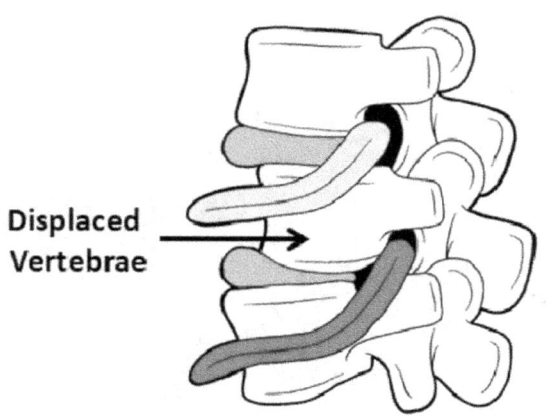

Figure 25 – Medical Subluxation.

According to the world of primary medicine, if you've got a medical subluxation, your problems are far worse than mine ever were. A medical subluxation is a serious medical condition that involves major structural damage. If you've got it, you are probably not walking and may never walk again. It would take a significant amount of force to create that kind of shift. This definition of a subluxation only applies to severe cases and the number of people suffering from the condition is very small.

Obviously, I don't have a medical subluxation condition. My MRIs never looked like the figure above. I've also never heard one person in primary medicine tell me that I had a subluxation. Now

I know why. According to medical science, a medical subluxation and a chiropractic subluxation are two very different things. Yet because chiropractic subluxations are relatively small and because imaging studies are only done on unloaded spines, they go undetected with X-Ray or MRI testing. And that confusion explains why millions of people, including myself, suffer for years and years with chronic back pain.

***

Primary medicine does not recognize the chiropractic definition of a subluxation and there's no medical term to describe a partial dislocation of the spine that is equivalent to the chiropractic definition. For that reason, no one in primary medicine believes that it is possible to dislocate the spine to a "small" degree; they are only looking for a large shift in the spine.

Yet the true cause of chronic back pain is a combination of very small shifts. That's all that is necessary to send a person into chronic pain. Thankfully, chiropractors physically look at the individual segments of the spine to determine if one vertebra is improperly rotated relative to another. If there were no chiropractors, millions more people would be living in chronic pain than there are today already. I probably wouldn't be alive today if it weren't for them, because they were my only source of pain relief for years and years.

It seems that most of the practitioners of primary medicine don't even understand what chiropractors actually do. They don't look at the spine directly; they are not trained to. Personally, no one in primary medicine looked at the individual segments of my spine. Every doctor that I have ever seen just did a nerve conduction test with a pinwheel or moved me into certain positions to try to recreate my pain. No wonder no one in primary medicine ever helped me.

Due to their disagreement about subluxation, one of these groups has to be wrong. Either everyone in primary medicine is wrong or every single chiropractor is wrong. If, as a policy, primary medicine doesn't believe that it's possible to only slightly dislocate the spine, then they are not going to see it as a medical problem, and they are not going to treat it. That's exactly what happened to me. The first time I hurt my back, I had a partial dislocation in my upper back. When I went to the Emergency Room in Glenwood Springs, they simply gave me pain medication and sent me on my way. When I was in Singapore, I happened to get lucky and correct my back's partial dislocation myself by bending over and spotting someone lifting weights. Once my subluxation went away, I was pain free.

The second time I hurt my back, I did not get as lucky. I had a subluxation in my lower back. I choose the route of primary medicine to help me, which was a big mistake. The healthcare system sent me to numerous doctors, orthopedic surgeons, physical therapists, and pain medicine specialists, all of whom considered the MRI to be the gold standard for revealing causes of problems. But because my MRI didn't reveal any significant subluxation in my spine, they told me nothing was wrong with my back. Because primary medicine does not recognize smaller subluxations as a problem—and cannot detect them with their expensive medical tests—my life was ruined. I spent years living with a dislocated spine. Besides being in pain, my ligaments were destroyed because I was never treated correctly. If I had not solved the cause of my back pain on my own, I would have taken it to my grave.

So how can I prove that primary medicine is wrong about subluxations? Well, it's actually very easy. Because primary medicine doesn't believe that a chiropractic subluxation exists, other groups have stepped up to fill the treatment void. There are over 100,000 chiropractors in the U.S. How do they stay in business? Clearly, they are providing a service that medical doctors won't and don't provide. They are treating non-major subluxations. While the medical community doesn't acknowledge that smaller subluxations exist, millions of people are suffering with chronic pain and paying hundreds of thousands of chiropractors to get temporary relief.

Check it out for yourself. Look up any city online and count the number of chiropractor offices that are listed. They are everywhere. I can throw a tennis ball from the yoga studio that I attend and hit a door to the office of three chiropractors. To get a sense of the number out there, let's just do some quick math. If there are 100,000 chiropractors in the U.S., they probably each need a minimum of 50 patients to stay in business. So that means that at least 5 million people across the country are seeing a chiropractor on a regular basis. My chiropractor is part of a low cost chain and they are open seven days a week. They must have well over 150 patients per chiropractor. Whatever the total number is, there are a lot of people out there who are seeing chiropractors!

If you walked into any chiropractor office, grabbed a patient who has a chiropractic subluxation that hasn't been treated, and took them to any hospital, the hospital would do a quick examination and take an X-Ray or MRI. Then they would find "nothing" wrong, give the patient painkillers, and send them home. Our only recourse would be to take the patient back to the chiropractor, who would treat the subluxation so the patient can finally go home pain-free. At least for a while.

Proof Positive

Consider that chiropractic care is commonplace and well-compensated in one big segment of our culture where it proves itself as a highly effective treatment: sports. Every professional sports franchise has a team chiropractor. Because the health of its players is crucial to the success of the team, sports franchises manage the health of its players independent of, and in addition to, mainstream healthcare. Since so much money is at risk, players are given any treatment necessary for them to perform at a high level. Their care includes chiropractic care; in fact, they may get adjustments before, during, and after a game if necessary. A subluxation is treated immediately when it occurs. Players don't have to go outside the franchise to have their subluxation corrected.

Yet, a regular person cannot walk into any hospital and have their subluxation treated. There are no chiropractors in hospitals. Something's definitely wrong for the rest of us who aren't professional athletes.

Chapter 11
Our Healthcare System

If you consider all of the procedures and therapies that I underwent to try to relieve my debilitating back pain as experiments providing key data points, then I should be able to analyze the data from those experiences and draw some sort of conclusion, or *correlation*. So, if my back pain decreased after trying a certain treatment, for example, I could conclude that the treatment worked. I certainly had seen enough practitioners to comprise a valid sample size.

If my experiments showed that primary medicine offered the most effective method to improve my health and reduce my pain, then a chart tracking the results would look something like this:

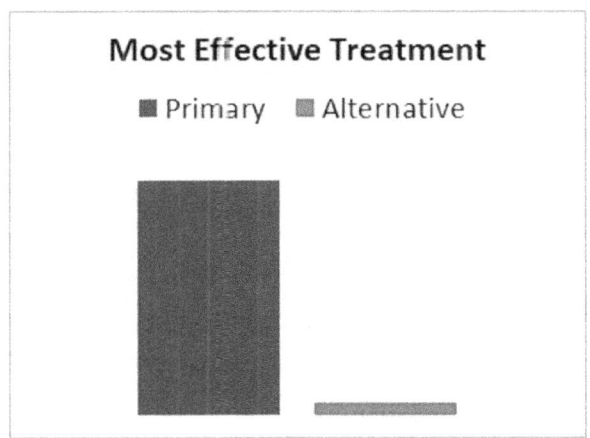

Figure 26

But in fact, every physical therapist I went to failed to help me and every surgery that I underwent failed to give me any long-term relief. Every nerve root block or epidural injection failed. The discogram failed. In fact, every procedure that primary medicine put me though failed me. Even though chiropractic was only providing temporary relief, it was significantly more effective than anything that primary medicine was offering.

That means that alternative medicine was by far the most effective treatment. My chart for it looks like this.

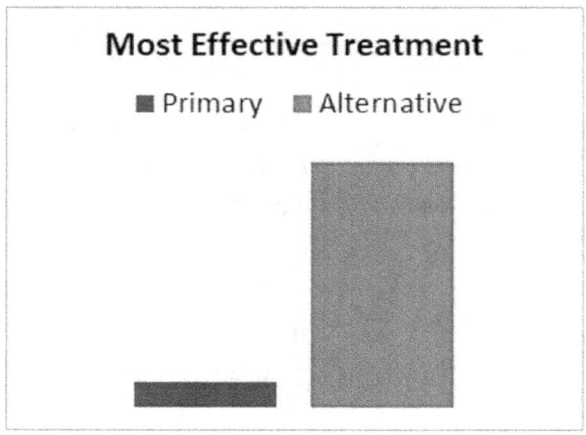

Figure 27

The results of my experiments revealed that primary medicine is not at all the most effective treatment for chronic back pain—yet it is unfortunately the standard treatment model for anyone suffering with it.

But here is where we run into a major problem, and it has to do with chiropractic care. Let's go back one more time and look at the definition of a chiropractic subluxation, according to Wikipedia.

In chiropractic, vertebral subluxation is a supposed misalignment of the spinal column leading to a set of signs and symptoms sometimes termed vertebral subluxation complex.

Notice the use of the word "supposed." It turns out that the definition for a chiropractic subluxation isn't taken very seriously. But there's more.

A 2009 review concluded that epidemiologic evidence doesn't support the existence of chiropractic subluxation, concluding:

"No supportive evidence is found for the chiropractic subluxation being associated with any disease process or of creating suboptimal health conditions requiring intervention. Regardless of popular appeal, this leaves the subluxation construct in the realm of unsupported speculation. This lack of supportive evidence suggests the subluxation construct has no valid clinical applicability."

The definition states that there is absolutely "no scientific evidence" to show that chiropractic care is an effective treatment for back pain. The treatment method apparently falls into the realm of "unsupported speculation" according to the write-up. But wait a minute! All of my experience and data conclude that chiropractic care was the most effective treatment for my chronic back pain—yet the definition claims that there is "no evidence to support" that it does anything at all. Really?

And, while there's "no evidence" to support the validity of chiropractic care, everyone's health insurance plan includes chiropractic care! Why? Either you believe in it or you don't. As we've discussed, there are over 100,000 chiropractors practicing in the United States. Every single professional sports franchise employs a chiropractor. Millions of people are seeing chiropractors regularly. And yet there is no evidence to support the need for chiropractic care at all? This is the state of our current healthcare system? It's an absolute joke. Why doesn't our healthcare include snake charmers and faith healers? It doesn't seem to matter that there is no evidence to support the validity of the methods they offer and cover.

Primary medicine doesn't recognize the chiropractic definition of a subluxation, yet our healthcare system has allowed a backdoor for people to receive chiropractic care. If a patient dislocates his spine, he must go outside a hospital to be treated because there are no chiropractors in any hospital. If there is no evidence to support the validity of chiropractic care, why let this practice exist?

Why No Scientific Evidence Supporting Chiropractic Care Exists

In order to answer this question, we have to look at the current healthcare model. The standard treatment model for someone who has hurt their back is, of course, to go to see their primary doctor. Turns out, the primary doctor knows nothing about back pain, so they will schedule an MRI, the gold standard for diagnosing back pain, and send the patient to a surgeon. If the MRI shows that there's nothing wrong and there's nothing worth operating on, then the conclusion is drawn that there is nothing wrong with the patient's back, regardless of how much pain they are in.

Since no one in primary medicine recognizes the possibility that the patient has dislocated their spine, the patient is not even checked for a misalignment. The patient has to deal with their subluxation on their own. One of the worst problems with this process is the time involved. By the time they get to a chiropractor, if they ever see a chiropractor, it is too late. The patient's ligaments have been destroyed. Their spine has become unstable from ligament laxity and almost any activity they participate in could potentially cause a subluxation. In other words, from that point forward, their life is ruined.

It's clear that all the studies and research that have been done to conclude that chiropractic care is useless were terribly flawed. Imagine trying to conduct a scientific experiment without knowing anything about ligament laxity. You put together a study that sends people with chronic back pain to a chiropractor to see if they can alleviate their pain. Of course, the chiropractor knows how to correct a subluxation, but they don't treat ligament laxity or muscle imbalance. That means it's only a matter of time before the patient's spine becomes dislocated again. Once the patient dislocates their spine again, they are back in pain. The only conclusion that could be drawn is that chiropractic care is absolutely useless because the patient requires repeated adjustments for life.

Hence, there's no scientific evidence supporting chiropractic care.

They only useful way to conduct an accurate study of chiropractic care would be to take a person who just dislocated their spine for the first time and send them to a chiropractor to treat it. Because the individual has no muscle imbalance issues and has not developed ligament laxity, scientific evidence will conclusively prove that chiropractic care is the most effective treatment for a dislocation. In fact, it is the only treatment. Once the patient is treated, they will never need another chiropractic adjustment ever again. The patient returns to their normal life.

This is why I put chiropractic care as the first step of my treatment method. If the flaws and errors in the current model to test the results of chiropractic care were eliminated, the results would easily demonstrate that a misaligned spine does cause pain and the spine must be placed back into alignment to relieve the pain before a treatment plan can begin.

Here is the sad part. Because whatever studies that were done to prove the validity of chiropractic care were done wrong, there are millions of people living their lives in horrible chronic pain. They are just ignored. Because primary medicine doesn't believe that it is possible for a person to dislocate their spine, there is a giant hole in healthcare. Primary medicine doesn't know what is wrong, much less how to treat it, so they just abandon everybody. Everything that chiropractors could have contributed to healthcare is ignored. In the meantime, the people in pain just get screwed.

Chapter 12
Why Chiropractors Get No Respect

When you walk into a chiropractor's office, the first thing they do is give you a canned speech about how chiropractic care will greatly improve your health because your spine will finally be in alignment. Their treatment model is that, with regular visits, your health will improve and at some point, you will be back to normal.

What they don't tell you is that the model only makes sense if it is the first time you dislocated your spine—and you don't have any of the other conditions that affect the dislocation, like ligament laxity issues, and muscle imbalance issues. You really only need one adjustment, but they we sell you on many more visits. Most of the people that have just dislocated their spine and get one adjustment become pain-free and don't return to the chiropractor.

They also don't tell you that if your spine was not treated properly the first time it was dislocated, you will require adjustment after adjustment for the rest of your life. You will never return to normal health. They know their treatment model is now crap, but it doesn't matter; they get paid every time you walk in the door. The more times you walk in, the more they get paid. The truth is that they have absolutely no idea what is wrong with you. They never tell you that they cannot solve your problem and return you to normal health. Therefore, they just treat you over and over and over again.

Flaws of Chiropractic Care

There are several factors that determine how effective a chiropractor is at correcting a subluxation. While it might sound like an easy process, it's not. When a person dislocates their spine, the asymmetrical neurological irritation drives their muscles into a super-tight state and the tight muscles pull their spine out of alignment. In order for a chiropractor to place the spine back into alignment, they have to overcome the force created by the muscles to create movement. If they cannot overcome the force created by the muscles, then an adjustment doesn't occur.

It's why a massage is often recommended before a chiropractic visit. Decreasing muscle tension increases the ability of the chiropractor to successfully correct a subluxation. But getting a massage before every adjustment can end up being very expensive and time consuming when continual chiropractic care is needed. For that reason, most people skip the massage and try to find a highly-skilled chiropractor.

A highly-skilled chiropractor understands how to manipulate the spine and remove subluxations. For this reason, loyalty is the heart of the chiropractic business. Once a person finds a skilled chiropractor, they will never go see anyone else. Even if they move, they will drive across town to see their chiropractor. People know if their dislocation is corrected. I knew exactly when I was in alignment and out of alignment.

So what happens when a patient goes to a chiropractor and doesn't get the proper treatment? The patient is left in pain. If the chiropractor cannot fix the subluxation, either through lack of experience, improper training, or extreme muscle tightness, then the patient walks out of their office with no solution to their pain.

The patient does not know if they've been treated properly since they are relying on the expertise of the chiropractor. If the patient is left in a subluxated state then their nervous system will be continuously irritated. They'll remain in that state until they go back to a chiropractor and hopefully get a proper adjustment. Many people experience chiropractic this way and then conclude that chiropractic care is useless because their problem never goes away. Instead of finding the right chiropractor, they just give up and live in chronic pain.

Another problem is that chiropractors are not created equal. Chiropractic colleges simply graduate as many people as they can and then let the market weed out the bad ones. When I told one of my chiropractors about my concern about this, he told me that he went to the "Harvard" of chiropractic colleges. There were 50 people in his graduating class, he told me, and out of those 50, he'd only let two or three work on his own spine. The colleges are doing a disservice to their own practice; there is absolutely no consistency among chiropractors. Patients rely on chiropractors for proper treatments but don't get it due to the lack of proper training of chiropractors.

Another reason chiropractors get no respect is that even if they are able to provide a proper adjustment, the patient's ligaments get completely destroyed. As a result, they have no stability of their spine. They could dislocate their spine just by getting up off of the chiropractic table or by getting into and out of their car. With such unstable patients, it becomes hard for chiropractors to be taken seriously since their patients constantly need more and more adjustments. The question is: Is it the chiropractor's fault or the patient's fault—or both?

It is also very interesting that even though chiropractic care is included in most everyone's health insurance plan, chiropractors have absolutely no medical stature. All records from chiropractors are disregarded. Their opinions have no value when it comes to making important medical decisions. Chiropractors thus serve no medical function.

The Solution

I think we are all in agreement that chiropractors are correcting dislocations of the spine. If there are 100,000 chiropractors in business out there, they must be providing a service of some sort. They must, at the very least, be providing temporary pain relief or they would not be in business. The problem is their placement in the overall treatment model. Chiropractors should be the first line of defense. If a person dislocates their spine and gets it treated immediately, the problem is easy to solve. One adjustment returns them to normal health. They will not fall victim to chronic back pain. But if they don't seek treatment immediately, all the other problems arise—ligament laxity, muscle imbalance, neurological irritation, short leg, and so on—and the problem becomes exponentially harder to solve. Then the other factors, like chiropractic skill level, become an issue. Because the issue of dislocation has grown into a problem of great complexity, the patient's chance of returning to normal health hovers near zero.

The solution to the problem is simple. Make chiropractors the first line of defense. Place a chiropractor in the emergency room. If we set up the system to treat patients immediately, chronic back pain will cease to exist. Better yet, train emergency room doctors to treat a dislocation of the spine. That way, both chronic back pain and chiropractors will cease to exist.

Chapter 13
How Physical Therapy Gets It All Wrong

When surgery is not an option, the most commonly prescribed therapies for those who hurt their back are physical therapy and chiropractic treatment. Beyond these two options, there are only a few additional choices left. One is pain management, which could easily result in an opioid addiction for the rest of the person's life, while it does nothing to solve their chronic back pain. Another option is steroid injections, which are completely useless for a person with ligament laxity. The last option might be to implant a stimulator in the spine. But that would only temporarily mask the pain.

Because I was in pain for so long, I saw a lot of doctors and surgeons. Even as they offered me no answers to resolve my back pain, they always gave the same advice: I should go to a physical therapist or a chiropractor. These are the fallback providers when primary medicine has no solution. Being a good patient, I listened to my doctors and surgeons, and I proceeded to go to physical therapist after physical therapist after physical therapist. I saw over fifteen physical therapists and every one of them failed me except the last one.

How could fifteen physical therapists fail to do any good? Let's dig into their treatment model.

The mantra you hear in physical therapy is all about strengthening your core. The assumption is that weak core muscles are the cause of back pain. Physical therapists tell you that if you strengthen your core, your back pain will go away and so they give their patients exercises to strengthen specific muscles. The expectation is that, when these exercises are done, they will eventually return to normal health sometime after their insurance has run out.

At first glance, their premise seems reasonable. It seems logical that if a muscle is weak and doesn't provide adequate support, then strengthening it will solve the problem. But that's a one-size-fits-all approach. Everyone is given the same treatment regardless of how strong their core was before they walked into the physical therapist's office.

Before I hurt my back, I was in awesome shape. I was very strong. I'd be in the gym doing crunches with a weight on my chest to make it even harder. Then I hurt my back, and a couple of months later, the physical therapist I was working with told me to do baby crunches with no weights because, she said, my core was weak. Was that a joke? It seemed absolutely insane to me that I could have a weak core. We have an entire field of healthcare that believes this huge generalization?

Now you might think that I was just lazy and I didn't do the exercises that were asked of me, and that's why the physical therapy didn't work time after time. But that's not the case. I loved to work out and I was extremely healthy before I hurt my spine. When I was given exercises to do, I far exceeded the amount and duration asked of me because I was living in chronic pain.

What's important to know, if you don't already, is that chronic pain is horrific. So I was open to anything that might provide even the smallest amount of pain relief. I did extra exercises because I was desperate for pain relief. I did everything they asked of me. Still, I experienced no improvement. Why had these physical therapists failed to help me? It was because my problem was structural.

Here's how the body works: The bones provide the structure to physically support the body. The ligaments provide the structural support for the joints, where two bones meet. The muscles provide movement for that joint. If a joint is dislocated, the ligaments become stretched and ligament laxity occurs. Once that happens, a joint is no longer stable. Because this instability occurs in the spine, the nervous system is irritated, causing pain and muscle tightness.

I had dislocated my spine and everyone in primary medicine failed to recognize it. My structural problem was due to ligament laxity that resulted from an undiagnosed dislocated spine. Strengthening core muscles cannot solve a structural problem. A person can triple the strength of their muscles and their ligament laxity problem will not go away. The only way to solve a structural problem is to fix the structural deficiency—which, in this case, is ligament laxity.

Here is how I think physical therapy got it wrong. A muscle can provide temporary structural support, but only if a muscle is contracted at the time it's needed to provide support. If you know you are going to get punched in the stomach, you can contract your muscles and lessen the impact. However, if you are punched in the stomach by surprise, you can't contract your muscles in time. The impact becomes far worse because all that force is transferred to your stomach. There is a reason fights are stopped when a person goes unconscious. Their muscles no longer provide any structural support and a punch can become deadly. When a person is unconscious, their ligaments provide the only structural support available.

When you go to the gym, you increase your muscle strength so you can lift more weight. But the second you put down that weight, your muscles go into a relaxed state. Our bodies are designed so that our muscles are not in continual use. The body only uses the minimum amount of force needed to maintain whatever position the body is in. When you stand, only the muscles needed to stand are recruited. When you lie down, no muscles are recruited. This is conservation of energy. Muscles were never designed to provide permanent structural support for the body. But ligaments were. That's why strengthening your core does nothing to treat ligament laxity — the real problem related to chronic back pain — and why physical therapists cannot and will not ever cure people with chronic back pain.

So, if muscles only provide temporary structural support, then why would a person want to strengthen them? Because if a muscle is injured or in the case of a subluxation, from neurological irritation, a muscle becomes weak. A weak muscle fatigues easily, which causes pain. The muscle can no longer do the task it was designed to do. Strengthening a muscle reduces its tendency to fatigue, thereby reducing the pain. The majority of people who have an injury never fully recover because they don't understand that a weak muscle must be strengthened to relieve pain.

The Physical Therapy Treatment Model

So why did physical therapy get it wrong? Physical therapy is called an "evidence-based" practice. That means that evidence shows that the majority of people achieve some sort of recovery with treatment. And, apparently, their treatment model works to some degree. But it clearly only works when it is used to treat some types of injuries. Not all.

The physical therapy treatment model makes perfect sense if the nervous system is not involved. If a person breaks their leg and the leg gets put in a cast, their leg muscles will become weak since those muscles aren't being used. Once the structural failure of the broken leg is fixed with the help of the cast, it makes perfect sense to then strengthen the muscles that have become weak. Their treatment model works perfectly in this kind of scenario. Almost everyone recovers from a broken leg.

However, their treatment model completely breaks down if the cause of the muscle weakness is due to a subluxation. A subluxation drives neurological irritation, which first creates muscle tightness and then eventually creates muscle weakness. A completely different treatment model than the broken leg model is needed to help this kind of condition. Every single physical therapist that I went to made the same assumption—that my weak muscles were the primary cause of my pain—and they ignored the true underlying cause: neurological irritation from a dislocated spine. And I was prescribed the same set of exercises over and over with the same result every time: no improvement.

Trying to strengthen a super tight muscle without removing the neurological irritation is insane. The only possible outcome of strengthening a tight, irritated muscle is to cause it to tighten up even more. Because no one understands how to properly treat the spine once a person hurts their back, it becomes a lifelong sentence. The recovery rate from chronic back pain is incredibly low. Just ask anyone with chronic back pain how effective physical therapy is as a treatment. You will be shocked to learn how many people try it and fail miserably. Every single person that I know who has chronic back pain got nothing from physical therapy, yet it remains the standard treatment model. The reason my last physical therapist was able to help me was because I removed my neurological irritation before I went to see him. With the irritation removed as a factor, strengthening and lengthening my weak muscles could correct my muscle imbalance. Fixing my ligament laxity problem enabled their standard treatment model to work. That's why my last physical therapist was finally able to help me.

The sad thing about our healthcare system is that physical therapy is the fallback therapy. If physical therapy, doesn't work, what is the patient supposed to do next?

Chapter 14
Categories of People

Now that you understand how chronic back pain works, we can categorize people into four groups.

Category 1

This is the group of people who live life without any experience of chronic back pain. They don't understand what a chiropractor does and have never needed to see one. Some might have seen a physical therapist for other issues besides the back. Some of the people in the group have never worked out or needed to stretch a muscle.

I lived in this category until the day I hurt my back.

Category 2

The people in this category have had a single instance of severe back pain. They might not know what caused their pain and most don't know what got it to go away. They were in severe pain and then the pain just went away. Perhaps they saw a chiropractor, maybe they had some other treatment, or perhaps they just moved a certain way and the pain completely disappeared. No one can explain to them why they were in pain or why it just magically went away. They weren't in pain long enough to call it chronic pain, and because the problem was corrected quickly, there was no permanent damage to their body. Their pelvis, shoulders, and neck remain level.

The first time I hurt my back, the pain simply, magically, went away after I bent over and lifted something.

Category 3

Folks in this category live with some form of chronic back pain every day. They have been forced to alter their lifestyle to deal with the pain and have learned other ways to manage it. They have figured out the signals that indicate that they need to go see a chiropractor to get a spinal adjustment. Whenever you hear someone say, "I threw my back out," they belong to this group. They are incredibly loyal to the one or two chiropractors who can give them relief from their pain because not all chiropractors can.

Because they were not given the correct treatment when they hurt their backs initially, the people in this category have ligament damage and so they need to get adjustments over and over and over again. If you were to examine any person in this group, you'd find that their head is leaning to one side. That's because if the ligament damage only occurs in the neck then their head will lean to one side. If their ligament damage occurs in their upper back, then both their shoulders and neck will be out of alignment. If the ligament damage occurs in the lower back, then their pelvis, shoulders, and neck will be off. Because of the existence of any of these conditions, their body will tilt to one side.

Every single person who has ligament damage in their lower back has a short leg. Depending upon where in their lower back the ligament laxity is, their sacrum may also have shifted. People with a shifted sacrum are easily identifiable. They can't sit down without being in pain.

Since, in the spine, everything is connected, it's very likely that when one area fails structurally, other areas of the spine will also soon fail. The individual might need to have adjustments done on different parts of their spine every time they go to a chiropractor.

Because this group has learned to manage their chronic back pain, they are probably not on painkillers or any other drugs for the long-term. But because their nervous systems are constantly being activated, they are burdened with muscles that are constantly tight. They might rely on massage or hot yoga to reduce pain. They might see a short-term gain with physical therapy since it helps to loosen muscles, but they won't see any long-term improvement.

I lived in this state until I learned to correct my ligament laxity problem.

Category 4

This group of people lives with severe chronic back pain every day. Every day is a struggle for them. These folks have the exact same problems as those in Category 3 but they don't know how to manage their pain. They have the identical ligament damage to their body but everything they have tried has failed. Physical therapy has failed them miserably. Either they don't believe in chiropractic care or they have tried it and didn't help. They may have tried multiple surgeries or injections, but they were all failures. Nothing is able to give them any relief from their severe pain. If they move the wrong way, they get a jolt of pain.

Their nervous system is constantly being activated and their muscles are incredibly tight. Even a massage provides very little relief.

Most people in this category either turn to pain medicine and other drugs to manage their pain, or they just live with the pain. They may have a stimulator implanted in their back as a last attempt to manage the pain and they might have been forced to severely alter their lifestyle just to get by. Most people in this category don't work or have a modified schedule; any kind of physical work is not an option. They feel like there is no hope and they have accepted that they will live in chronic pain until they die. Since no one in healthcare understands the cause of their pain, they are abandoned by their healthcare system. It's easy to identify the individuals in this group just by looking at their faces. They are incredibly unhappy. A certain percentage of the people in this group die every year either from taking their own life or from an accidental overdose of the painkillers they are living on every day.

I lived in this state until I learned how to manage my pain with chiropractic care.

Something in Common

The last three categories of people all have something in common: a single event changed their lives. Some are forever changed and will live in chronic pain for the rest of their lives. Others have a miraculous recovery where the pain just goes away. Either way, they will never forget the day that they hurt their back. The event is so traumatic that, years later, even those who are now pain-free remember when they had horrible back pain.

So how big of a problem is ligament laxity? As far as Category 3 people are concerned, they usually rely on chiropractic care to keep them out of pain. From that, we can conclude that they are free from pain from time to time. The fact that they achieve a pain-free state proves that there is no significant disease causing their pain. This rules out all diagnoses given by doctors because people in Category 3 can get their pain significantly reduced with nothing more than a spinal adjustment. With that understanding, we can conclude that 100% of the people who see chiropractors on a regular basis have a ligament laxity issue. One could also argue that if ligament laxity didn't exist, there would be no need to go to a chiropractor—ever. It's actually easy to prove. A normal, healthy person never goes to a chiropractor, ever. There is no need. No ligament laxity means no spinal adjustments are needed.

Category 4 people are a little harder to diagnose. But one thing stands out about them. If you look at their posture, you can see it. For most of the people in this category, their shoulders are not level, and that's an indication ligament laxity. They were misdiagnosed and so they were never treated properly. Considering posture alone, you'd probably be right to conclude that their back pain is due to ligament laxity.

That leaves a very small group of people who have an underlying issue that's different from everyone else. It may be a genetic defect or the presence of a growth. It might be visible on an MRI and might require surgery. It could also be the result of having multiple failed surgeries. Once a person has had multiple surgeries and hardware implanted in their spine, determining the cause of their pain is near impossible. Normal treatment methods, like chiropractic care, provide absolutely no pain relief. If you add up all of the people who fall into this group, the number is incredibly low.

Because everyone in primary medicine believes that if a dislocation of the spine isn't significant enough to appear on static imaging studies, then it doesn't exist, these people's lives are changed forever. Often, they're completely ruined. How can it stand that millions of normal and healthy people endure a single event that leaves them in chronic pain for the rest of their life? Why does primary medicine have no solution for them?

Chapter 15
Other People With Chronic Back Pain

Once I learned how to identify and fix my own body's structural issues, I was able to look at other people and determine what structural issues they had, too. I was absolutely amazed at what I discovered, namely, other peoples' bodies had failed in the same identical way that my body had failed. All bodies fail in a similar manner.

Since then, I've become a posture expert. I can look at someone and be able to tell if they have a leg-length discrepancy. The interesting thing is that once you start looking, you find that there are a lot of people with short legs out there. They are easy to spot. Anyone with a short leg has uneven shoulders, their head leans to one side, their pelvis is tilted, and their gait is off. And they complain of the exact same pain that I complained of.

I would like to introduce you to a few people I've met who have some level of chronic back pain. Understanding their conditions will help you put together all the pieces of what I've been talking about. I don't use their real names, but I will personally introduce you to them if you desire.

***

I begin with my brother. My brother started having horrible back pain, so I took him to the same chiropractor that helped me diagnose my short leg. It turns out he had short leg, too, but with the opposite leg. Because we were able to identify the cause of his pain, we were able to dramatically change his life with just a heel lift. What was interesting about his situation was that his quadriceps had become so tight that his gait was affected. His gait was more of a prance than a stride.

Of course, even though my brother's back pain went away, his muscles didn't automatically return to normal function. Because of that, he still doesn't have a normal gait. He's a perfect example of the principle that, even if back pain is no longer a problem, the muscles need to be lengthened to return them to normal function. He is among the Category 3 people. He occasionally uses a chiropractor to manage his pain.

**

My neighbor also has chronic back pain. He now has an electrical stimulator implanted in his back so that he can manage his pain. It's easy to see that his shoulders and head are not in alignment—he obviously has a short leg. Yet what's amazing to me is that his symptoms almost matched mine exactly. He has lower back, upper back, and neck pain, as I did. We both even have TMJ issues from our necks leaning to one side. It's also interesting that he fits into both Category 3 and Category 4. He learned how to adjust his upper back on his own, but he could not figure out how to adjust his lower back or neck. He does not use chiropractors to manage his pain and so some parts of his spine are always out of alignment. Just a little bit of a wrong movement gives him a jolt of pain. He medicates if he needs to do physical work. He continues to work, but his life has been severely altered.

**

A friend of a friend had stopped working because of the chronic pain she constantly suffers from. She hurt her back from an incident on an airplane, fits into Category 4, and lives on painkillers every day. Everything she tried has failed, including physical therapy. One day, she called me up and asked if I would meet her at her chiropractor's office the next time she went, to see what I thought. When I arrived there, I immediately knew why she was getting no relief from her treatment, but I kept quiet and waited to hear what the chiropractor had to say. He had taken a full length X-Ray and had drawn lines on it to show how far out of alignment her pelvis was. To me, it was blatantly and ridiculously obvious from everything I saw—in her stance and in the X-Ray film—that this woman had a short leg.

But it was what the chiropractor did next that really shocked me.

Instead of giving her a heel lift and taking a new X-Ray showing her pelvis was moved into alignment, the chiropractor just said, "Let's wait and see what the MRI shows." The chiropractor did not understand that my friend had a short leg and so he didn't treat her for the condition that was really the problem. I was stunned that the chiropractor would let her walk out of his office with an untreated short leg. This poor woman would be left to deal with her chronic pain on her own.

My friend's pain is identical to what mine was. She has neck, upper back, lower back, and sacrum issues, as I did. She also lost her ability to sit down without being in excruciating pain. She will live on painkillers until she dies.

***

I met a woman in a yoga class who stopped working because of chronic pain that started after she was in an automobile accident. I actually showed her how far off her pelvis, shoulders, and head were. When I gave her a wearable posture lift and a heel lift to try, she immediately felt better. But someone told her not to use those devices, so she stopped using them. Her pain is also very similar to what mine was. Sitting down for her is as brutal as it was for me. She uses chiropractic to manage her pain but she is in too much pain to work. She fits into Category 3. Her lifestyle has been severely limited. She will live in chronic pain until she dies.

***

A relative of mine has been on disability for a very long time. His shoulders are not level, indicating a short leg. He is a Category 3 type and uses chiropractic to manage his pain.

***

Another friend of mine has some very interesting issues. He can sit all day long, but standing is very painful for him. I've only met two people that have that set of conditions. One thing that is different about him is that his shoulders are never level, even when he is in alignment, because of a huge self-inflicted scoliosis. I had taken a look at his chiropractic records and I was stunned by what I found. His spine had failed in the exact same places that my spine had failed.

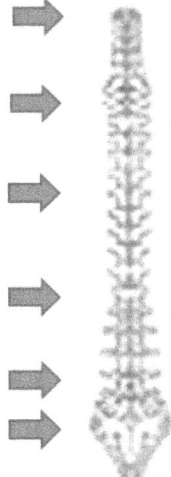

Areas Of The Spine Prone To Subluxation

Figure 28 *Remember this?*

His neck, upper-back, lower-back, and sacrum all had areas that were prone to subluxate. He would have to get all of those areas checked every time that he went to see a chiropractor. This is scientific proof that a short leg unevenly loads the spine causing other areas of the spine to fail.

The only difference between my spine and his spine is that his sacrum shifted on the side with the short leg, while my sacrum had shifted on the opposite side of my short leg.

His approach to solving his back pain was to seek out the "very best"—but even the very best physical therapists could not fix his back problem. He is in Category 3, uses a heel lift, and gets chiropractic adjustments and massage to manage his pain.

***

During the time that I was designing a wearable posture lift, I met the owner of a specialty shoe store who would give my product to people for me. I just wanted to see if other people would get the same results that I got. One person he gave it to came back to the store a year later, and he was still using the product. He would wear it anytime he had to be in a car for a long period of time. This was proof that his sacrum had shifted in exactly the same way mine did. We both got the same amount of relief from placing our sacrum back into alignment. He is in Category 4 because he does not see chiropractors, but just deals with the pain on his own. His life has been severely altered because of chronic back pain.

***

I can go on, naming one person after another who has chronic back pain but is not getting any relief from it. How many more stories do you need to hear? I could probably describe at least thirty people who I know personally with chronic back pain. What do all of these people and millions of other people have in common besides pain? They all look like this.

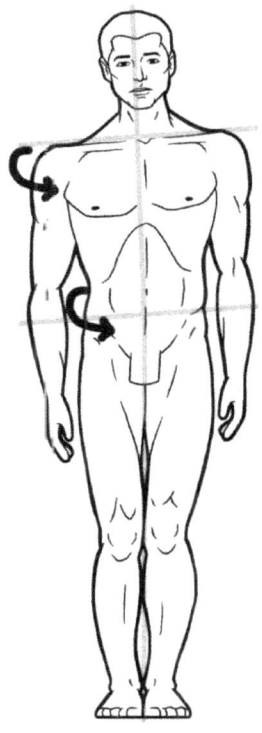

Figure 29

They all have a short leg. That means they all have ligament laxity. What else do these people have in common? They have all been abandoned by their healthcare system. There was no easy surgery option and physical therapy failed them, so they are left to live the rest of their life with chronic pain. Why aren't teams of specialists trying to solve this problem? These are real people, in pain, begging for help.

When someone hurts their back, it's reasonable to think that one area of their spine would be in pain. But most people with chronic pain complain of pain in several areas of their back. They have some combination of pain in their neck, upper back, lower back, and possibly even sacrum. How is this possible? I posed that question to a physical therapist. His response was to say that "everything is connected." Not much of an answer. And he never could answer specifically why the other areas of the spine were also in pain. The reason that he couldn't answer the question was because primary medicine does not recognize that a subluxation of the spine is possible if it doesn't show up on their tests. Without the understanding that a subluxation causes the spine to tilt, which unevenly loads the spine, which in turn causes other areas of the spine to subsequently fail, he could not properly answer the question.

He did not understand that one untreated structural problem can mushroom into many more structural problems.

Chapter 16
I Can Ruin Anyone's Life

The beauty of science is that once a hypothesis is proven, it can be tested over and over again and still produce the exact same results. The methodology that was used to solve the original problem can be used to solve other problems—or to replicate the original problem. Now that I've deduced the cause of chronic back pain, not only can I help people, I can also hurt them. I can choose to use my powers for good or evil.

Because of the years I spent scientifically investigating the cause of my own chronic back pain; I now have enough information to cause enough chronic pain in people that they will never be able to work again. With my help, they'd never have one pain-free day as long as they live.

With that in mind, I want to put a study together. The people in the study would include physical therapists, neurologists, spine surgeons, chiropractors, massage therapists, and pain medicine specialists. I'd also run the study on the people who are responsible for running the business side of healthcare, like administrators and insurance plan providers. Lastly, I would include the judges who are responsible for disability claims. Anyone who is over 40 in the study will make it go more smoothly.

Here's what I'd do with the participants in the study. First, I'd give them a heel lift and a wearable posture lift. The combination would cause a short leg. Because of their short leg, their pelvis would lower and be tilted forward on the side with the short leg. The heel lift would ensure their pelvis gets rotated when they are standing. The wearable posture lift would ensure that the pelvis is rotated while they are sitting and lying down. These correction devices wouldbe used to keep the pelvis in a rotated state.

Soon enough, a muscle imbalance issue would occur. Some muscles would get overused while other muscles would not be needed and would be underused.

Everyone's new short leg would cause their gait to be off. Their short leg would swing further and hit the ground differently with every step. Even simply walking would require their body to compensate in some way for every step they take. Muscles that are not normally used would become overworked. With every step, their short leg would also drive their pelvis out of alignment.

Because of their new short leg condition, their bodies would lean to one side. Their shoulders and neck would no longer be in alignment and that misalignment would no longer load the spine evenly. The areas of the spine that carry more of the load would tend to rotate out of alignment. Because of *proprioception*, our ability to instinctively understand the position of our body parts, their heads would want to be in an upright position, but they wouldn't be able to because of the misalignment. Some of their neck muscles would become overworked. Their body would slowly adapt to the misalignment caused by the short leg. Their ligaments would be put under strain.

These factors alone may not cause any pain right away, but their bodies would be set up for failure.

The next step would be to create a subluxation. Chiropractors apply a force to rotate the spine back into alignment. I would just reverse the process: applying enough force to cause a subluxation. It is simple physics. I'd rotate one part of the body in one direction and another part in the opposite direction, and increase the force until the joint is dislocated. I'd only need to dislocate the spine by a very small amount to irritate their nervous systems.

Once I created the subluxation, the life of everyone in the study would change dramatically. They would be in pain 24 hours a day. Their short leg would be much shorter. Their body's alignment would be off by the amount of the heel lift plus the amount of the subluxation. The dislocation would cause their nerves to be irritated asymmetrically and their muscles would clamp down in response to the irritation. The positive feedback loop they have entered into would drive a muscle imbalance issue.

The final thing I'd want to do in the study would be to leave the participants in a dislocated state—which happens to be exactly what primary medicine does to the rest of us anyway. Everyone's ligaments would quickly become destroyed. Even if the subluxation or the muscle imbalance were corrected, their ligaments would remain damaged forever. Every single movement they make would need to be evaluated as to whether or not it would cause more pain. Every participant in the study would finally understand the pain that millions of people, including myself, have been living with every day. They, too, would have to learn to live with chronic back pain.

What happens next would be something of a snowball effect. Because one leg has become much shorter than the other, their spines would be way out of alignment. Their shoulders and necks would be off even more. The uneven loading of the spine would cause more vertebrae to dislocate. The more vertebrae that dislocate, the greater the leg length discrepancy becomes. Yes, a Catch-22. Then, every vertebra that gets dislocated destroys its neighboring ligaments.

When the ligaments of so many vertebrae are damaged, the chances of at least one of them having a subluxation are substantially increased. How do you even approach treating someone with ligament laxity in three, four, or five different areas of the spine? The problem of chronic back pain becomes exponentially harder to solve.

Now you know why people who have back pain are condemned to live with it until they die. The sad part is that some of the people in this study will end their lives. After years and years of searching for someone to help them, once they realize no one can, they will lose all hope and cease to exist.

If I were able to complete such a study, I'd find one thing very interesting. If I were to disable a social security judge then I'd prove that the entire healthcare system is wrong. After all, such a judge has been making legal decisions based on the direction of the healthcare system. Once I prove the healthcare system is flawed, the judge's decisions would all become invalid. The entire system would need to be revamped.

If you think for one second that anything I've written in this book is inaccurate, I encourage you to take part in my study. In fact, I'm begging you to take part in the study. See for yourself what happens to your own body when you dislocate your spine. Once you live with chronic back pain for a while, you will have a new understanding of the hell that people with chronic back pain live with every day.

No Takers

I worked with a physical therapist for almost nine months trying to solve my muscle imbalance issues. We discussed in great lengths the ideas that I've presented in this book. One of the topics we discussed was leg length discrepancy. He told me that he believed, as all physical therapists believe, that a person can have a leg length discrepancy of up to one inch without experiencing any pain or other issues. (He commented, "I know that sounds like a lot.") He clearly does not understand how a short leg condition affects the body and how it spirals into chronic back pain. Yet he is among the professionals that we all should be able to count on to be posture specialists.

It is absolutely crucial that physical therapists identify and treat short legs. If they do not treat a short leg, no one else will. There is no one else in the entire healthcare system that even treats posture.

In order to demonstrate to my physical therapist what a short leg does to the body, I invited him to be a part of my study. I could easily prove that any leg length discrepancy is bad, let alone the one-inch discrepancy that all physical therapists believe is not a problem.

My plan was to start him off wearing wear a heel lift to create a short leg. We would start with a standard heel lift of 3/8th of an inch. Then we'd slowly increase the size of the heel lift to one inch. Since he was only 28 years old, there was a very good chance that his body would adapt to the heel lift and not cause any major issues. However, he would start to endure some pain. He would start to understand that his gait was getting disturbed and his feet were no longer contacting the ground correctly. When he walked, muscles that he didn't normally use would become overworked and tighten up. His pelvis would shift and his entire spine would begin to lean to one side, causing more muscles to tighten. His neck muscles would also tighten. I do not even need to dislocate his spine for him to understand how a short leg dramatically affects the body. He would soon learn what his patients with short legs were enduring.

My goal was to explain to him that a leg length discrepancy of any size was bad, but a one-inch leg length discrepancy was insane. I knew we could use the information to change the treatment model of physical therapy forever. He would have firsthand knowledge of it.

What he did next shocked me. He refused to test it out with me. He said, "I do not know what this is going to do to my body, so I would rather not do it." He also said, "I do not have time in my life to be bothered with this."

These are the people in healthcare who are responsible for treating people with postural issues and they do not even want to learn how posture affects the body. They allow their patients to have a leg length discrepancy but they sure as hell do not want one. Shouldn't these people at least practice what they preach? I guess as long as you are not the one in pain, nothing else matters.

Chapter 17
How Did I Get Here?

Why did I have to solve my chronic back pain problem on my own? There was clearly a disconnect in the system that allowed millions of people like myself to slip through the cracks and not get proper treatment. I wanted to know why. I wanted to sit down with the people on the front lines of healthcare for chronic back pain.

So I started with physical therapists.

I had met a physical therapist at a poker table who was two years out of college and had a Ph.D. It was perfect. I figured that a recent graduate should be up-to-date on the latest thinking and techniques for treating chronic back pain. He hadn't worked on a lot of chronic back pain patients but he had been trained to work on them.

Over the next several months, we discussed the topic of subluxations in great detail while he helped me fix my muscle imbalance issues. I gave him a thorough explanation of how I dislocated my spine and I described to him how, due to the fact that it had not been treated correctly, a ligament laxity condition had developed. He read my book and understood how I arrived at the conclusions I came to. He decided to do some research into the physical therapists' official position on a subluxation and discovered that they do have a definition for a subluxation, but they call it a "bone out of place." Their position is that it is possible for a bone to be out of place in the spine and it may possibly cause pain, but, they claim, it is "a very rare event." He told me that according to their professional reference materials, "the structures of the spine prohibit a dislocation or a subluxation from occurring."

When I asked him about treating a "bone out of place," he told me that physical therapists do treat them. Now, I have seen a lot of physical therapists and I have never ever had one treat my dislocated spine in a similar way to the way chiropractors treat them. I knew he was bluffing, so I tested him. Because his office was right next door to a chiropractor's office, I said, "If you treat subluxations, let's go to the chiropractor's office and you show me how you treat it."

He replied, "Well you cannot expect me to do what they do. They have years of training!" He refused to demonstrate his point. His actions were proof that physical therapists weren't only untrained in recognizing subluxations, they were also never trained to treat them.

So I dug deeper.

"If physical therapists acknowledge that a dislocation of the spine is possible, then shouldn't the standard treatment protocol dictate that a patient with a dislocation or subluxation be treated immediately?" I asked.

"Yes," he responded.

"Well, since physical therapists aren't trained to treat subluxations, shouldn't the patient be referred to someone who does treat them?"

"Yes."

"But as of right now, physical therapists are not treating subluxations and they are not referring their patients to anyone else that can treat them either, right?"

"Right."

It's very confusing. Physical therapists believe that it's possible for someone to dislocate their spine, but claim it's a very rare event. At the same time, there are over 100,000 chiropractors that do nothing but treat a "bone out of place," day in day out, year after year. In fact, it's their only treatment method. So we can easily conclude that a subluxation is not a rare event at all.

Clearly, somebody's getting it wrong. When I brought it up to the physical therapist, he ended our conversation. He didn't want to talk about it anymore. This is what he believed and he was not willing to listen to anything different or consider another position.

Orthopedic Surgeons

The next group I wanted to speak to was orthopedic surgeons. They are the first ones that the medical community refers to when someone hurts their back.

Coincidentally, when I was in the casino talking to the physical therapist, a woman sat down next to us. Overhearing our conversation, she started laughing. She told us that she was an orthopedic surgeon and she joined our conservation about chronic back pain. We talked for over an hour and I asked her a lot of questions.

"What do you think is the cause of chronic back pain?" I asked her.

"Some people are obese and that could be the cause the chronic back pain," she said.

I asked her to show me one study that positively correlates obesity to chronic back pain. She did not have a response.

"Do you have any other ideas about causes of chronic back pain?"

She didn't answer. I kept expecting her to give me some direct answers for the cause of chronic back pain, but I never got them. It was as if she did not know how to answer my questions—but she was the one doing the surgeries!

But she did tell me that she absolutely hates operating on the spine. The chances of a positive outcome are so low, she said, that she would rather not operate. She said that if she helps one out of four people, she feels successful. She also said something interesting about her profession. She said she thought it was truly amazing that some surgeons will continue to operate on people with chronic pain who have already failed multiple surgeries, even though they know the potential outcome of a successful surgery is incredible low. They continue tooperate on people, as if the next surgery will be some sort of a miracle surgery. It baffled her. She knew enough to know that any further surgery was useless.

Then she admitted something. She said that if orthopedic surgeons cannot figure out what is wrong with a patient, they send them to physical therapy. This explains why I was sent to so many physical therapists. Because I was in horrible chronic pain, I went to orthopedic surgeon after orthopedic surgeon. Because there was nothing obvious on my MRI, and so there was no obvious surgery for them to do, they just sent me to one physical therapist after the next. After I failed physical therapy, I was sent back to an orthopedic surgeon until they found something to operate on. Then I was sent back to a physical therapist again. Like me, millions of patients are sent through this endless loop of healthcare until either they run out of money or they just give up because they realize that no one is going to help them.

What baffles me is the fact that these are highly educated people we are talking about. If treatments of surgery and physical therapy are consistently failing people, why isn't someone speaking up? Shouldn't they at least inform the medical institutions that educated them? They watch the system fail people over and over again and they do nothing about it. They can have a lifetime's worth of failed patients but no one seems to care.

In the almost 20 years since I first hurt my back, absolutely nothing has changed. If someone injures their back today, they will go through the exact same rat hole I went through. Sure, some of the surgeries are a little different and some of the physical therapy techniques are a little different. But every day, people are walking into emergency rooms with dislocated spines and they are not being treated. They are sent home with painkillers. The basic treatment model is exactly the same as it was 20 years ago.

Why Did I Have to Solve This Problem?

In order to better understand why there was no help for me, we have to look at how our healthcare system works. Providers are guaranteed payment before any patient walks through the door. Since they are guaranteed payment, there is no reason to ever deviate from what they have been taught. If the patient does not improve, it is not their fault. They are doing exactly what they were taught. They won't ever get in trouble if they do exactly what they were taught. Patient outcomes mean absolutely nothing. If they fail patient after patient, it does not matter. The patient can die and they still get paid.

Because of the way the system is set up, there is absolutely no innovation. Even though they are highly educated people, they have no reason to change. If you look at other monopolies, you will see the exact same business model. There is very little innovation because they do not need it. Because they are guaranteed payment, healthcare providers have no reason to innovate.

From the outside, the healthcare system looks like a well-oiled machine. Even though I received absolutely no pain relief from countless providers, I guarantee you that my medical records indicate something entirely different. The reason is because the people who were treating me were also the ones that were updating my medical records, and it would be insanely stupid for them to show that they are incompetent. For example, my medical records state that my level of pain went from 9 to 1 after my artificial disc surgery. That's a lie. I experienced nothing of the sort.

Once you start peeling back the layers, you see a very different reality. There are millions of people who are going to chiropractors because no one in primary medicine will help them. Ask any one of them why they do not go to the hospital when they hurt their back and everyone will tell you the same thing: it is a complete waste of time and money to go to a hospital. They tried it and the system failed them. At least chiropractors provide them with temporary relief.

How to Solve Chronic Back Pain

Here's my solution to eliminating chronic back pain everywhere almost completely. It is very simple. It is called forced innovation. The solution is to tie provider pay to patient outcomes. The patient would be treated and then given some amount of time after treatment to see if they have actually improved. If the patient doesn't improve, the provider does not get paid. It's that simple.

If this were enacted, we'd see a mass exodus from everyone working on chronic back pain. If the providers don't get paid, they will stop working on the spine. They will immediately shift to other parts of the body. If surgeons are not completely sure that they can provide a good outcome, they will not operate. All of these useless surgeries will cease to exist. Physical therapists will only treat body parts that they know will heal. Chiropractors will go out of business because their treatment model is based upon repeated adjustments.

What makes this solution especially beneficial is that, after the mass exodus, the few remaining providers who are left would be forced to innovate and to actually find a solution to chronic back pain. They would have to seek out help from anyone who might help them solve the problem, even people like me because I have at least presented a solution for chronic back pain. Any idea would have to be investigated. The beauty of this approach is that once chronic back pain is solved, no one ever has to suffer from it ever again. This is the beauty of science. Once a problem is solved, the solution can be applied to everyone.

The worst problem with the current healthcare system is that the patient has no voice. People with chronic back pain do not fit neatly into a single category that is easily solvable, so they are abandoned. There is not even a single person who manages the health of chronic pain sufferers. If such a person existed, they would have easily seen how horrendously awful the current healthcare system is. There are millions of people with horrible chronic pain and it does not matter.

I Did It My Way

I was left to solve the problem of chronic back pain on my own. I was able to solve the problem because I looked at the problem differently than everyone else does. Because of flawed thinking from primary medicine, my body was never once evaluated as a structure. Yet the body is a structure and when a structure fails, there is a root cause for the failure. I was able to take what I needed from each provider and also incorporate my own ideas to solve my structural problem. Once I did this, my chronic back pain went away.

So why was no one able to solve this problem? Chronic back pain is a complex problem. The solution requires people to take a number of steps in the correct order to achieve the proper outcome. If these steps are not followed correctly, the process fails. Our healthcare system is not set up to solve complex problems; it is set up to treat problems individually. Solving individual components can never solve a complex problem. A single provider could never solve the chronic back pain problem by themselves. Providers work independently of each other. In fact, they do not even talk to each other and that makes problem-solving incredibly difficult.

So let's look at what each provider does. Chiropractors only treat subluxations or dislocations of the spine. They do not treat muscle imbalance or ligament laxity. Physical therapists only treat muscle imbalance. They do not treat dislocations or ligament laxity. Orthopedic surgeons try to solve structural problems through surgery by either removing something or adding something. They do not treat muscle imbalance or dislocations. They might treat ligament laxity indirectly through a fusion or by adding hardware, but they do not treat ligament laxity directly. Pain medicine specialists only address neurological irritation that results from structural failure. They do not treat muscle imbalance, dislocations, or ligament laxity. PRP doctors use injections to treat ligament laxity. They do not treat dislocations or muscle imbalance.

If a representative from each of these groups of providers were to sit down and have a conversation about chronic back pain, they might actually solve the problem. Individually, they have nothing. Together, they comprise the solution. That's how I ended my debilitating back pain: I got what I needed from each discipline in a way that got me the result I was seeking.

Starting the Conversation

At the beginning of this book, I presented the hypothesis that the current method for treating chronic back pain is fundamentally flawed. I did so because people are hurting their backs and are never able to recover from it. That truth didn't make sense to me. If a person breaks their arm, for example, they have a near 100% chance of recovery. But when it comes to back pain, providers don't how to treat it, and patients never recover. There is no other explanation. Making matters worse, they don't admit that they don't know how to treat the problem, they ignore it, and they force their patients to repeat unsuccessful treatments for the rest of their lives.

I wrote this book to start a conversation. The current treatment protocol for chronic back pain is not working. Anyone that works in healthcare and watches patient after patient fail to recover can attest to that fact. Or, ask anyone with chronic back pain and they will tell you that they have had nowhere to turn because no one knows how to help them. They will tell you they feel abandoned by their healthcare system. Ask them how it feels to be in pain all day long. Ask them why their life is a living hell. Start asking questions. If chronic back pain is ever going to be solved, someone has to start a conversation.

Even better, assemble a team of open-minded individuals who actually want to solve the chronic back pain epidemic. Let them figure out why so many people never recover. Let them determine the cause of chronic back pain. They will come to the same conclusion that I did. Chronic back pain is caused by a structural failure of the spine.

Now, I have presented a treatment method to drastically alter people's lives. But I have a problem. I am not in medicine; I am only an engineer. So the only thing I can do is present my ideas. I can't change the system on my own. I need help.

Please help me change the system and let's help the millions of people who are suffering. There is an opportunity to significantly change medicine forever.

There is one thing I can do. If you are living with chronic back pain, I can show you how to get your life back. I can show you the process that I went through and I can introduce you to the people who I think will be most beneficial for your return to normal health. You have read my story. If I was able to fix my back, then I can definitely help you fix your back. The only way I can change the system is to start helping people. If I can help one person, then writing this book was worth it. If I can help thousands of people, I can change the course of medicine forever.

Chapter 18
Living Pain Free

For over 16 years, I felt like a dog that was beaten over and over and over again. I felt powerless to stop the chronic, horrific pain and no one was able to help me, either. I didn't have one pain-free day in all of those 16 years. When I look back at how much pain I was in, part of me is shocked that I am still alive. There were many, many days when I wasn't sure that I would be able to make it through the day.

Then one day, the torture stopped and my life began to change. Once I learned what was wrong with me, things started to take a different direction. As I began to solve problem after problem, things got better. But I had to dig myself out of a gigantic hole. Through trial and error, along with a lot of hard work, my life changed even more. Here are the most important things that are radically different in my life thanks to all the work I did:

I no longer see a chiropractor. I had multiple areas of my spine that needed constant adjustment. I always had at least one area that was out of alignment, leaving me in constant pain. My spine was so unstable that I could not do anything without the fear of dislocating it. Now, I do not need any chiropractor adjustments at all. I have not had an adjustment on any part of my spine in over a year, and it's been over two years for certain areas of my spine. I don't see any reason why I would ever need to go back to a chiropractor again.

I do not need any posture correction. My pelvis was rotated so far out of alignment that I needed constant correction to help calm down my nervous system. Just to stand up without any correction was painful. Sitting down was horrendously painful. I would have to change positions very frequently. Sit. Stand. Sit. Stand. Over and over. Now, my spine is perfectly straight. My pelvis, shoulders, and head are level. I can sit for hours now, completely pain-free.

I do not need any medication. While I was never a fan of taking drugs to mask pain, when I first hurt my back, I spent several years trying different drugs to alleviate my pain. I was scared to death of becoming an opioid addict, so I preferred to live in pain rather than take that chance. Every drug left me in a fog and I hated it. Now, I am so grateful that I do not have to take any medications, ever. There is no pain to mask.

My quality of life has skyrocketed. I was the type of person that loved to be very active but chronic back pain stole all that from me. I never wanted to get off the couch. Every aspect of my life changed drastically. Now, I am resuming the activities that I once loved. I work out at the gym almost every day. I am getting stronger every day. I play golf pain-free and I hike for hours.

I still have a little bit of a beaten dog syndrome. I hope that the "person" that was beating me never comes back. I am cautious. I watch what I do and how I do it. I will never play contact sports again or do some of things that I did when I was younger, but that's okay. The risk is not worth the reward. I have made major strides in lengthening and strengthening my muscles. I know which of my muscles have issues and I know how to address them to keep myself functioning at a high level.

I now enjoy a quality of life of about 9. Compared to where I have been, it is a monumental improvement. Every day, I seem to feel a little better. I have gotten my life back. Every day is a great day.

Contact the author at

chronicbackpainsolved@gmail.com.

www.ingramcontent.com/pod-product-compliance
Lightning Source LLC
Chambersburg PA
CBHW071539220526
45469CB00003B/851